HEALING WITH SOMATIC EXERCISES

10 MINUTE ROUTINES TO REGULATE YOUR NERVOUS SYSTEM - RELEASE TRAUMA, STRESS, ANXIETY, AND ACTIVATE YOUR VAGUS NERVE TO BALANCE YOUR MIND-BODY CONNECTION

J.C MYLES

Copyright © 2025 by J.C MYLES

All rights reserved.

No portion of this book may be reproduced in any form without written permission from the publisher or author, except as permitted by U.S. copyright law.

This publication is designed to provide accurate and authoritative information in regard to the subject matter covered. It is sold with the understanding that neither the author nor the publisher is engaged in rendering legal, investment, accounting or other professional services.

While the publisher and author have used their best efforts in preparing this book, they make no representations or warranties with respect to the accuracy or completeness of the contents of this book and specifically disclaim any implied warranties of merchantability or fitness for a particular purpose.

No warranty may be created or extended by sales representatives or written sales materials. The advice and strategies contained herein may not be suitable for your situation. You should consult with a professional when appropriate. Neither the publisher nor the author shall be liable for any loss of profit or any other commercial damages, including but not limited to special, incidental, consequential, personal, or other damages.

First edition 2025

CONTENTS

Introduction	v
1. Foundations of Somatic Healing	1
2. Preparing for Your Somatic Practice	11
3. Gentle Movements for Chronic Pain and Muscle Release	19
4. Body-Focused Healing for Trauma and PTSD	33
5. Calming the Nervous System for Anxiety Relief	45
6. Overcoming Depression and Low Energy	57
7. Stress and Burnout Recovery Through Mind-Body Techniques	67
8. Restoring Gut Health and Digestion Naturally	79
9. Better Sleep Through Deep Relaxation and Breathwork	93
10. Support Immunity and Reduce Inflammation Through Body Awareness	103
11. Integrating Somatic Practices into Daily Life	115
Conclusion	123
References	127

INTRODUCTION

A few years ago, I met a woman named Sarah who had been carrying a heavy burden of trauma and stress for most of her life. She had tried various therapies and medications, yet nothing seemed to provide lasting relief. One day, she stumbled upon somatic exercises. She was skeptical at first, but she decided to give it a try. Over time, she noticed profound changes. Her body felt lighter, her mind clearer, and she began to feel a sense of peace she hadn't known in years. Sarah's story is just one of many that illustrate the transformative power of somatic exercises.

So, what exactly are somatic exercises? Simply put, they are a type of body-focused practice designed to help you become more aware of your physical sensations and release stored tension. Unlike traditional exercises that focus on strengthening muscles or improving cardiovascular health, somatic exercises aim to connect the mind and body. They are particularly effective for addressing trauma, stress, and emotional tension because they work directly with the nervous system.

The purpose of this book is straightforward. I want to help you release trauma, stress, and emotional tension stored in your body.

INTRODUCTION

Following the practical exercises outlined in this book can boost your mind-body connection and improve your overall well-being. Each chapter focuses on specific conditions, providing actionable exercises to address issues like chronic pain, anxiety, depression, and more.

This book is for everyone. Whether you are young or old, a beginner or an experienced practitioner, you will find value in these exercises. They are designed to be accessible and effective for people of all ages who are looking to release trauma, stress, and emotional tension stored in the body.

The book's structure is designed to guide you through various aspects of somatic exercises. Each chapter focuses on a different condition:

- Chronic Pain and Physical Tension
- Trauma and PTSD Recovery
- Depression and Low Energy
- Stress and Burnout
- Digestive and Gut Health
- Sleep Improvement
- Immune System Support and Inflammation

Allow me to share a bit about myself. My name is J.C Myles, and I am passionate about helping people overcome trauma, stress, and emotional tension stored in the body. With years of experience in this field, I have worked with countless individuals to help them achieve a stronger mind-body connection.

The effectiveness of somatic exercises is backed by scientific research. Studies have shown that these practices can help regulate the nervous system, reduce symptoms of PTSD, and improve overall emotional well-being. This book draws on this research to

INTRODUCTION

provide you with exercises that can make a real difference in your life.

I want to encourage you as you begin this journey. You have the power to transform your life through these exercises. Approach them with an open mind and a commitment to your well-being. Remember, the healing journey is a marathon, not a sprint. Take it one step at a time, and know that every small effort brings you closer to a healthier, more balanced life.

So, let's get started. Dive into the chapters, try out the exercises, and feel the changes in your body and mind. The path to healing is in your hands.

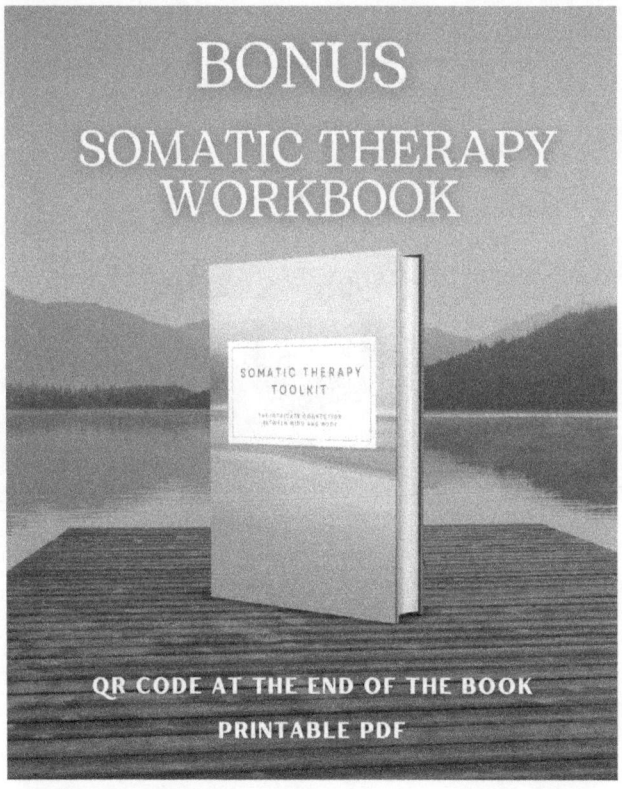

INTRODUCTION

At the end of chapters three to ten, you'll find a QR code linking to video classes designed to guide you through the somatic exercises

CHAPTER 1
FOUNDATIONS OF SOMATIC HEALING

SCIENTIFIC FOUNDATIONS OF SOMATIC THERAPY

Somatic exercises aren't just new-age hype; they are grounded in robust scientific research. Numerous studies validate their efficacy, particularly for trauma and stress-related conditions. For instance, a review of the literature up to August 2020 found that Somatic Experiencing (SE), a body-oriented therapeutic approach, has significant positive effects on PTSD-related symptoms, emotional well-being, and even physical health. This review analyzed 16 studies that met rigorous criteria, underscoring the growing evidence base for somatic practices.

The findings are compelling. For example, a study published in the Journal of Traumatic Stress reported that veterans who practiced somatic exercises experienced notable reductions in PTSD symptoms and stress levels. Another study highlighted that somatic practices can reduce chronic pain, offering relief where traditional methods often fall short. This research collectively underscores the potential of somatic exercises to bring about meaningful change.

The neurophysiological mechanisms behind somatic exercises are equally fascinating. One key concept is neuroplasticity, the brain's ability to reorganize itself by forming new neural connections. Somatic exercises leverage this by helping the brain "relearn" how to interact with the body, promoting healthier responses to stress and trauma. The longest nerve in your body also plays a big role. This nerve, which extends from the brainstem to the abdomen, regulates the parasympathetic nervous system—the part of the nervous system in charge of rest and digestion. Stimulating the vagus nerve through specific somatic exercises can activate this calming system, reducing stress and enhancing emotional regulation.

Experts in the field lend further credibility to these practices. Dr. Peter Levine, the developer of Somatic Experiencing, emphasizes that somatic exercises help individuals process trauma through the body's natural healing mechanisms. "Our bodies are equipped to heal if we allow them to," he often says. Dr. Bessel van der Kolk, a renowned trauma researcher, echoes this sentiment. In his book "The Body Keeps the Score," he writes about the transformative power of body-focused therapies, stating, "Trauma victims cannot recover until they become familiar with and befriend the sensations in their bodies."

In clinical settings, somatic exercises are increasingly integrated into therapeutic practices. Physical therapists use them to help patients manage chronic pain, enhancing traditional treatments with body-focused techniques. Mental health professionals incorporate somatic exercises to help clients process trauma and regulate their emotions. These examples show the versatility and effectiveness of somatic practices in both physical and mental health contexts.

CHAPTER 1

UNDERSTANDING SOMATIC EXERCISES

Somatic exercises are not your usual gym routine or a yoga class. They are body-focused practices designed to help you become more aware of your physical sensations and release stored tension. These exercises are particularly effective for trauma, stress, and emotional tension because they work directly with the body's natural healing mechanisms. Unlike traditional exercises focusing on muscle strength or cardiovascular health, somatic practices aim to reconnect the mind and body. This approach allows you to process and release the stress and trauma stored in your muscles and tissues, allowing you to destress your body and mind.

The origins of somatic practices are rooted in various traditions and disciplines. While the concept of mind-body integration has been present in ancient healing practices, the modern approach to somatic exercises has been influenced by fields such as psychology, neurology, and physical therapy. Early pioneers like Thomas Hanna and Moshe Feldenkrais developed methods that emphasized body awareness and gentle movements to enhance physical and emotional health. These foundational ideas have evolved, giving rise to a variety of somatic modalities that we see today.

Physically, somatic exercises offer numerous benefits. They can significantly reduce pain and manage chronic conditions by focusing on releasing tension and improving body alignment. Enhanced flexibility and mobility are other key advantages. As you become more attuned to your body, you'll likely notice an increase in overall physical awareness, which can help stop injuries and improve posture. For instance, after a long day at the office, gentle stretches can alleviate the tension built up in your neck and shoulders, providing immediate relief and promoting long-term health.

The mental and emotional advantages are just as compelling. Somatic exercises are powerful tools for managing stress, anxiety, and emotional tension. Techniques like breathwork can instantly calm your nervous system, making it easier to handle stressful situations. Building emotional resilience is another crucial aspect; as you practice, you'll find it easier to deal with life's challenges with a sense of balance and calm. For example, using breathwork during a stressful workday can help you stay centered and focused to reduce the stress on your mental health.

Different types of somatic exercises cater to various needs. Breathwork focuses on controlled breathing techniques to calm the mind and body. Body scans guide you through a mental check of your body, helping you identify areas of tension. Gentle movements and stretches improve flexibility and release physical stress. Visualization techniques use mental imagery to promote relaxation and emotional healing. Each type has its unique benefits, and incorporating a mix can provide a well-rounded approach to somatic healing.

Real-life applications of somatic exercises are endless. Imagine using breathwork to calm your nerves before a big presentation at work. Or performing a body scan before bed to prepare for a restful night's sleep. Gentle stretches can be a lifesaver after hours spent hunched over a computer. These practices can easily integrate into your daily routine, providing immediate benefits and contributing to long-term well-being.

THE SCIENCE BEHIND THE MIND-BODY CONNECTION

The concept of the mind-body connection is foundational to understanding somatic exercises. At its core, the mind-body connection refers to the intricate and dynamic interplay between our mental states and physical sensations. This connection is significant because it illustrates how our thoughts, emotions, and physical experiences are deeply intertwined. When we experience stress, for

CHAPTER 1

instance, it's not just a mental event; our bodies respond with increased heart rates, muscle tension, and other physiological changes. Recognizing this interconnectedness is crucial for effective somatic practice.

Scientific research has increasingly validated the importance of this connection. One study found that somatic exercises significantly aid in trauma recovery. Participants reported fewer PTSD symptoms and an enhanced sense of well-being. Another research highlighted in the journal Frontiers in Psychology showed that somatic practices could reduce stress and improve emotional regulation. These studies collectively affirm that engaging the body in specific ways can lead to profound psychological benefits.

The physiological mechanisms underlying the mind-body connection are complex but fascinating. The nervous system plays an important role in this interplay. When we practice somatic exercises, we engage both the central and peripheral nervous systems. The vagus nerve, which connects the brain to other important organs, is particularly important. This nerve influences the parasympathetic nervous system, which is responsible for relaxation and recovery. By stimulating the vagus nerve through somatic exercises, we can activate this calming system, reducing stress and enhancing our emotional resilience.

Somatic exercises also influence brain activity. Research has shown that these practices can boost neuroplasticity, letting the brain form new neural connections. This is particularly beneficial for people recovering from trauma, as it helps the brain "relearn" healthier responses to stress. For example, a study in NeuroImage demonstrated that somatic practices could lead to increased brain activity in areas associated with emotional regulation and less activity in areas linked to stress responses.

The practical implications of these scientific insights are substantial. Improved emotional resilience is one of the most significant benefits. By regularly practicing somatic exercises, you can develop a stronger ability to handle emotional challenges, reducing the impact of stress on your daily life. Enhanced physical health is another key outcome. As you become more attuned to your body, you'll likely experience less chronic pain and better overall functionality. Effective stress management is yet another advantage. With these exercises, you can quickly and efficiently calm your mind and body, making it easier to navigate stressful situations.

HOW SOMATIC EXERCISES AFFECT THE NERVOUS SYSTEM

Somatic exercises and the nervous system share a delicate dance that reshapes your body's responses and fosters healing. When you engage in somatic exercises, you tap into the brain's remarkable ability to change—known as neuroplasticity. This concept explains how the brain can form new pathways and reorganize itself. By practicing specific movements and techniques, you encourage your brain to create healthier patterns, transforming how you process stress and trauma. Imagine your brain as a garden, where somatic exercises are the tools that help you prune away the weeds and cultivate flourishing plants.

Mechanoreceptors and proprioception also play crucial roles in this process. Mechanoreceptors are sensory receptors in your skin and other tissues that respond to touch, pressure, and movement. Proprioception, on the other hand, is your body's ability to sense its position and movements. These receptors send signals to your brain, helping it understand what's happening within your body. Practicing somatic exercises enhances these sensory pathways, making your brain more attuned to your body's needs. This improved awareness can lead to a reduction in chronic pain and improved nervous system regulation.

CHAPTER 1

Activating the parasympathetic nervous system is another key aspect. This part of your nervous system is responsible for the "rest and digest" functions, promoting relaxation and recovery. Somatic exercises often emphasize slow, deliberate movements and controlled breathing, which stimulate the vagus nerve—a critical component of the parasympathetic system. Doing so can downregulate the sympathetic nervous system, which is associated with the "fight or flight" response. Achieving this balance between the sympathetic and parasympathetic systems reduces stress and fosters long-term health.

Nervous system regulation is all about maintaining this delicate balance. When your sympathetic and parasympathetic systems are in harmony, your body can efficiently manage and recover from stress. Techniques like progressive muscle relaxation and slow, deliberate movements are designed to help achieve this balance. For example, progressive muscle relaxation requires tensing and slowly releasing different muscles, which can help calm your nervous system and reduce anxiety. The long-term benefits of such balanced regulation include improved emotional resilience, better sleep, and a more robust immune system.

To illustrate these concepts, let's look at some specific exercises. Vagus nerve stimulation techniques, such as deep diaphragmatic breathing and cold water face immersion, are highly effective. These practices can quickly activate the parasympathetic nervous system, promoting relaxation. Slow, deliberate movements like Tai Chi or gentle yoga stretches can also help regulate your nervous system, making you feel more centered and calm. As mentioned earlier, progressive muscle relaxation provides a structured way to release tension and foster a state of relaxation.

Scientific research supports these effects. Studies on neuroplasticity have shown that somatic exercises can lead to improvements in brain activity, promoting healthier emotional responses. Research on chronic pain relief indicates that these practices can reduce pain intensity and improve quality of life. Evidence supporting stress reduction highlights the potential of somatic exercises to lower stress hormones and enhance overall well-being. These findings collectively underscore the transformative power of engaging with your body in mindful, intentional ways.

COMMON MISCONCEPTIONS AND MYTHS DEBUNKED

When it comes to somatic exercises, a few common misconceptions can cloud our understanding and discourage people from trying them. One prevalent myth is that somatic exercises are just like yoga. While both practices involve the body and mind, they serve different purposes. Yoga often focuses on flexibility, strength, and mental peace through structured poses and sequences. On the other hand, somatic exercises aim to release the tension and trauma stored in the body through more subtle, individualized movements and awareness. They don't require you to hold challenging poses or follow a set routine; instead, they encourage intuitive, mindful engagement with your body.

Another common myth is that you must be flexible to benefit from somatic exercises. This couldn't be further from the truth. These exercises are designed to meet you where you are, regardless of your physical condition or flexibility level. The goal is not to stretch your body to its limits but to cultivate an awareness of your bodily sensations and release stored tension. Even small, gentle movements can have profound effects. For instance, simply rotating your shoulders or practicing deep breathing can bring noticeable relief and relaxation. Flexibility is not a prerequisite; awareness and intention are what matter most.

A third myth suggests that somatic exercises lack scientific backing. This misconception likely comes from a lack of widespread knowledge and occasional misrepresentation in the media. However, numerous scientific studies support the efficacy of somatic practices. For example, a review published in the Journal of Traumatic Stress highlights the positive impact of somatic exercises on PTSD symptoms and overall well-being. Experts like Dr. Peter Levine and Dr. Bessel van der Kolk have extensively documented the benefits of body-focused therapies in their research and clinical work. These endorsements provide robust evidence that somatic exercises are indeed grounded in science.

Encouraging an open-minded approach is crucial for first-time practitioners. It's easy to dismiss something unfamiliar, especially when it challenges conventional wisdom. However, the potential benefits are immense. Many people find unexpected relief from chronic pain, improved emotional resilience, and a deeper connection to their bodies. Imagine starting your day with a simple body scan and ending it with a few minutes of mindful breathing. These small practices can accumulate, significantly improving your overall well-being. Keeping an open mind allows you to fully explore the possibilities and discover what works best for you.

In conclusion, somatic exercises are distinct from practices like yoga, do not require flexibility, and are backed by solid scientific evidence. By dispelling these myths, we can open the door to a more informed, accessible, and practical approach to healing. Approach these exercises with curiosity and an open heart. You might be surprised at the profound changes you experience.

CHAPTER 2
PREPARING FOR YOUR SOMATIC PRACTICE

CREATING A SAFE PRACTICE ENVIRONMENT

Imagine walking into a room that instantly makes you feel relaxed. The lighting is soft, the air is fresh, and there's a gentle hum of calming music in the background. This is the type of environment that can significantly enhance your somatic practice. A quiet and distraction-free area is crucial. This isn't just about physical safety; it's about creating a mental and emotional sanctuary. When you're distracted by external noises or interruptions, focusing on the subtle signals your body sends you is hard. Find a place where you can close the door and tune out the world for a while. This could be a spare room, a section of your bedroom, or even a quiet spot in your backyard. The key is choosing a space where you feel secure and fully immerse yourself in the practice.

Lighting and ventilation are also essential elements. Natural light is ideal, but soft, adjustable lighting can work wonders too. Avoid harsh, fluorescent lights that can strain your eyes and make you feel tense. Good ventilation ensures that the air is fresh and that you're not breathing in stale or stuffy air, affecting your ability to relax. Open a window or use a fan to keep the air circulating and pleasant.

Privacy is another critical factor. Knowing that you won't be interrupted allows you to let go and focus entirely on the exercises. This might mean scheduling your practice time when others in your household are out or preoccupied. If privacy is hard to come by, consider using a room divider or curtain to create a semi-private space.

Setting up your practice space can be a delightful experience. Start with soft flooring or a yoga mat to provide cushioning and support. This protects your joints and encourages you to move freely without discomfort. Comfortable seating options like cushions or bolsters can make seated exercises more pleasant. Think about the colors and decor in your space. Calming colors [blues, greens, and earth tones] can create a soothing environment. Add elements that make you feel good, like plants, soft blankets, or inspiring artwork.

The ambiance of your practice space plays a significant role in your experience. Soft, adjustable lighting can help set the mood, making it easier to relax and focus. Consider using dimmable lamps or fairy lights to create a gentle, inviting glow. Sound is another powerful tool. Calming music or nature sounds can drown out background noise and help you stay present. Platforms like Spotify or YouTube offer countless playlists and tracks explicitly designed for relaxation and meditation. Aromatherapy with essential oils can also enhance your practice. Scents like lavender, chamomile, and sandalwood are known for their calming effects. Use a diffuser or a scented candle to fill your room with these soothing aromas.

Creating a safe space can be challenging if you have limited room or a busy household, but it's entirely possible with a bit of creativity. Temporary setups in small apartments can work just as well. Roll out a yoga mat in your living room, or use your bed as a practice space. Portable props like small cushions, foldable mats, or even a travel diffuser can make it easier to practice on the go. Scheduling quiet time is another strategy. Communicate with your household members about your need for uninterrupted practice time. You might find that early mornings or late evenings are perfect for finding that quiet.

ESSENTIAL TOOLS AND PROPS FOR SOMATIC EXERCISES

Starting with a yoga mat or soft flooring can make a world of difference. A yoga mat provides the cushioning and stability needed for many somatic exercises. It protects your joints, making it easier to move and stretch without discomfort. If you don't have a yoga mat, consider using a thick towel or blanket to create a soft surface. This can be especially useful for exercises that involve lying down or sitting for extended periods.

Supportive pillows or bolsters are another must-have. These tools offer comfort and support during exercises that require you to hold positions for a while. For instance, when practicing deep breathing or gentle stretches, a pillow can support your back or neck, allowing you to relax more fully. If you don't have specialized bolsters, regular bed pillows or even rolled-up towels can work just as well. The goal is to find something that provides enough support to keep you comfortable and focused on the practice.

Stretch bands or resistance bands are excellent for enhancing stretches and adding a bit of resistance to your exercises. These bands can help you achieve deeper stretches and improve your range of motion. They are particularly useful for exercises targeting specific muscle groups, like the shoulders or hips. If you don't have resistance bands, you can use old tights or leggings as a DIY alternative. The elasticity of these items can provide similar benefits, allowing you to get the most out of your stretches.

Investing in high-quality tools can significantly enhance your somatic experience. A premium yoga mat, for example, offers better durability and comfort than cheaper alternatives. It's less likely to wear out quickly, providing a stable and comfortable surface for your practice. Similarly, ergonomic props like specialized bolsters or cushions are designed to support your body in the most effective way. These tools can make your practice more enjoyable and sustainable, encouraging you to stick with it over the long term.

For those on a budget, there are plenty of creative alternatives. Towels or blankets can serve as makeshift mats, providing a soft surface for your exercises. Household items like chairs or books can be used as props for various exercises. For instance, a chair can support you during standing stretches, while a stack of books can serve as a makeshift bolster. The key is to be resourceful and use what you have to create a comfortable and supportive environment.

The benefits of investing in quality tools go beyond just comfort. High-quality tools are designed to help you get the most out of your practice. A good yoga mat, for example, provides the right amount of grip and comfort, making it easier to maintain stability during exercises. Ergonomic props are specifically designed to support your body, reducing the risk of strain. These tools can make your exercises more effective, helping you hit your goals more quickly and efficiently.

While practicing somatic exercises with minimal equipment is possible, having the right tools can enhance your experience and make it more enjoyable. Whether you invest in high-quality props or use budget-friendly alternatives, the key is to create a comfortable and supportive environment that lets you focus on your practice. This will set you up for success as you work to release trauma, stress, and emotional tension stored in your body.

CHAPTER 2

UNDERSTANDING AND RESPECTING YOUR BODY'S LIMITS

Understanding your body's limits is crucial for a safe and effective somatic practice. It starts with recognizing the difference between pain and discomfort. Pain is your body's way of signaling that something is wrong and should be addressed immediately. It can feel sharp, burning, or stabbing and usually indicates an injury. Discomfort, on the other hand, might feel like a dull ache or tightness and can be a normal part of stretching and moving muscles. Listening to these bodily signals helps you distinguish between pushing your limits safely and causing harm. When you feel pain, stop the activity and reassess. When you feel discomfort, proceed with caution and awareness.

Practicing safely is about more than just avoiding pain; it's about creating a sustainable routine that promotes long-term well-being. Warm-up exercises are a great place to start. These activities prepare your muscles and joints for more intense movements. Simple actions like gentle stretching, walking in place, or doing light yoga can effectively warm up your body. Gradual progression in intensity is another key factor. Start with simpler, less demanding exercises and slowly increase the intensity as your body adapts. This approach allows your muscles and joints to adjust, minimizing the risk of overuse injuries. Proper alignment techniques are also critical. Ensuring that your body is correctly aligned during exercises can prevent strain and enhance the effectiveness of your practice.

Modifications and adaptations are essential for making somatic exercises accessible to everyone, regardless of their physical condition or experience level. Adjusting poses to suit your flexibility levels can make a significant difference. For instance, if a full stretch is too challenging, try a modified version that still provides benefits without straining your muscles. Using props for support can also help. Items like pillows, blocks, or straps can make exercises more comfortable and achievable. These tools can assist in maintaining proper alignment and reducing the risk of injury. Alternative exercises for specific conditions are also important. If a particular movement is too painful or difficult, find a substitute that targets the same muscle group but in a way that suits your body's needs.

Rest and recovery are often overlooked but are vital components of any exercise routine. Your body needs time to heal and rebuild after physical activity. Adding rest days into your routine allows your muscles to recover, reducing the risk of overtraining and burnout. Signs of overtraining include persistent fatigue, decreased performance, and increased susceptibility to injuries. Paying attention to these signs can help you adjust your practice and prevent long-term damage. Sleep and nutrition also play crucial roles in recovery. A good night's sleep lets your body repair itself, while proper nutrition provides the fuel and building blocks for muscle recovery and overall health.

Recognizing and respecting your body's limits is not a sign of weakness but an intelligent approach to long-term health and wellness. By listening to your body, practicing safely, making necessary modifications, and allowing adequate time for rest and recovery, you create a sustainable practice that supports your overall well-being. This mindful approach ensures that your somatic exercises are both practical and enjoyable, helping you release trauma, stress, and emotional tension stored in your body.

THE IMPORTANCE OF CONSISTENCY IN SOMATIC PRACTICE

Consistency in somatic practice is crucial for long-term success and transformation. When you engage in these exercises regularly, you allow the benefits to accumulate and create lasting change. Building habits through repetition is the key here. Just as brushing your teeth daily keeps your mouth healthy, regular somatic practice keeps your body and mind balanced. Over time, these small, consistent actions lead to positive enhancements in both physical and mental health. Imagine the difference between watering a plant daily versus sporadically; the same principle applies to your well-being.

The long-term benefits of maintaining a consistent practice are numerous. Physically, regular somatic exercises can lead to improved flexibility, reduced pain, and better posture. Mentally, they can help manage stress, improve emotional regulation, and enhance overall well-being. Regular practice trains your nervous system to respond more calmly to stressors, making it easier to navigate life's challenges. Think of it as building a reservoir of resilience that you can draw upon in times of need.

Staying committed to a regular routine can be challenging, but there are several strategies to help you maintain consistency. Scheduling dedicated practice times is one practical approach. By setting aside specific times for your somatic exercises, you create a habit and make it a non-negotiable part of your day. This could be as simple as dedicating ten minutes every morning or evening to your practice. Creating accountability with practice partners can also be motivating. Sharing your goals with a friend or being part of a somatic exercise group can provide the support and encouragement you need to stay on track. Setting reminders and alerts on your phone or calendar can serve as helpful prompts to keep you on schedule.

Common barriers to consistency include time constraints and lack of motivation. Life gets busy, and finding the time for self-care can be challenging. One way to manage time constraints is by integrating somatic exercises into your daily routine. For example, you can apply deep breathing exercises while driving or do gentle stretches during your lunch break. Dealing with a lack of motivation requires a bit of creativity and self-compassion. On days when you feel unmotivated, remind yourself of the benefits you've experienced so far. Sometimes, starting with just a few minutes can lead to a longer session once you get into the flow.

Consistency in somatic practice is not just about repetition but about creating a sustainable routine supporting your long-term health and well-being. By understanding the importance of regular practice, employing strategies to stay committed, overcoming common barriers, and drawing inspiration from others, you set yourself up for success. The benefits of consistent practice are profound, offering you the tools and resilience needed to navigate life's challenges with greater ease and grace.

CHAPTER 3
GENTLE MOVEMENTS FOR CHRONIC PAIN AND MUSCLE RELEASE

RELEASING NECK TENSION WITH GENTLE STRETCHES

Neck tension is a frequent complaint for good reasons. The neck is a complex muscle structure that bears the weight of your head, a hefty 10-12 pounds, all day long. When you're stressed, your body often responds by tightening these muscles, exacerbating the problem. Poor posture, whether hunched over your computer or craning your neck to check your phone, can worsen matters. This combination of stress and poor posture creates a vicious cycle of tension and pain.

Gentle neck stretches can be incredibly effective in breaking this cycle. Let's start with a simple but powerful exercise, **Side-to-Side Neck Stretches**:

1. Sit comfortably with your back straight.
2. Calmly tilt your head to the right, bringing your ear toward your shoulder.
3. Hold for a few seconds, then return to the center.

4. Repeat on the left side.

This stretch helps release tension in the sides of your neck and improves flexibility.

Another effective stretch is the **Forward and Backward Tilt**:

1. Begin in the same comfortable seated position.
2. Gently lower your chin toward your chest, feeling the stretch along the back of your neck.
3. Hold for a few seconds, then lift your chin and tilt your head back, stretching the front of your neck.

This movement helps counteract the forward head posture many of us develop from prolonged sitting and screen time.

Neck Rotation Exercises are also beneficial:

1. Sit or stand with your back straight.
2. Calmly turn your head to the right, looking over your shoulder.
3. Hold for a few seconds, then return to the center.
4. Repeat on the left side.

This exercise helps extend the range of motion in your neck and helps release tension. You can use a towel or strap to enhance these stretches. For example, during the side-to-side neck stretch, gently pull on the towel to deepen the stretch. This modification is particularly helpful if your neck muscles are very tight.

If you prefer to perform these stretches seated, ensure your back is well-supported. Sit on a chair with a backrest, or use a cushion to support your lower back. This position helps maintain proper alignment, making the stretches more effective. Alternatively, you can perform these stretches standing, which engages your core muscles for stability.

To modify these stretches for different levels of flexibility and comfort, consider using props like a towel or strap. If you find reaching your shoulder during the side-to-side stretch challenging, loop a towel around your head and gently pull it toward your shoulder. This modification allows you to control the intensity of the stretch. For the forward and backward tilt, you can perform the exercise seated or standing, depending on what feels more comfortable for you. If you're seated, ensure your back is well-supported to maintain proper alignment.

Incorporating these gentle neck stretches into your daily routine can significantly reduce tension and pain in your neck. This practice improves your physical well-being and enhances your overall quality of life. Remember, the key is consistency. Regularly performing these stretches will help you maintain a healthy, flexible neck, making it easier to manage stress and enjoy daily activities without discomfort.

ALLEVIATING LOWER & UPPER BACK PAIN WITH SOMATIC MOVEMENT

Back pain is a common issue that many people face daily. Several factors contribute to this discomfort, including a sedentary lifestyle, poor lifting techniques, weak core muscles, and stress. Sitting for a long time can lead to tightness in the lower back, while improper lifting can strain muscles and ligaments. Weak core muscles fail to support the spine adequately, leading to imbalances and pain. Stress and tension exacerbate these issues, causing the muscles to tighten and creating a cycle of discomfort. Specific somatic movements can be highly effective in addressing lower back pain.

Pelvic Tilts are a great starting point:

1. Lie on your back.
2. Bend your knees and keep your feet on the floor.
3. Slowly tilt your pelvis upward, flattening your lower back against the ground, then release.

This movement helps to mobilize the lower back and reduce tension.

The **Cat-Cow Stretch** is another excellent exercise:

1. Start on your hands and knees.
2. Alternate between arching your back like a cat and dipping it like a cow.

This dynamic movement increases flexibility and alleviates stiffness.

Child's Pose is a calming stretch that gently elongates the lower back:

1. Kneel on the floor.
2. Sit back on your heels.
3. Extend your arms forward.
4. Lower your chest to the ground.

Finally, the **Supine Spinal Twist** is perfect for releasing tension:

1. Lie on your back.
2. Bring one knee toward your chest and let it fall across your body.
3. Keep your shoulders flat on the floor.

This twist helps to decompress the spine and release tight muscles.

CHAPTER 3

For upper back relief, shoulder blade squeezes, and thoracic spine rotations work wonders.

To perform **Shoulder Blade Squeezes**:

1. Sit or stand with your back straight.
2. Squeeze your shoulder blades together.
3. Hold for a few seconds.
4. Release.

This exercise toughens the muscles between your shoulder blades, improving posture and reducing tension.

Thoracic Spine Rotations are also beneficial:

1. Sit with your feet flat on the ground and place your hands behind your head.
2. Slowly rotate your upper body to the right, hold, and then rotate to the left.

This movement increases mobility in the upper back and helps to alleviate stiffness.

Strengthening your core muscles is vital for preventing lower back pain. The deep core muscle engages the transverse abdominis and provides stability to your spine. Core stabilization exercises like planks and bridges are excellent for this purpose.

For **Planks**:

- Hold your body in a straight line from head to heels.
- Engage your core throughout.

For **Bridges**:

- Lie on your back with your knees bent.

- Keep your feet flat on the floor.
- Lift your hips toward the sky.
- Squeezing your glutes and engaging your core.

These exercises build strength and support for your lower back.

A structured daily routine can significantly improve back pain management if you are consistent:

- Start your day with a **morning** stretch sequence to wake up your muscles and warm up your body for the day ahead.
- **Midday** mobility exercises can prevent stiffness from prolonged sitting. Incorporate simple movements like shoulder rolls and seated twists to keep your back flexible.
- An **evening** relaxation routine can help you wind down and release any accumulated tension. Gentle stretches and deep breathing exercises are perfect for this time of day.

Integrating breathwork and mindfulness into your somatic movements enhances their effectiveness. Coordinating your breath with movement keeps you present and aware during exercises. For example, inhale deeply as you prepare for a stretch and exhale slowly as you move into the stretch. Staying present and aware helps you connect with your body, ensuring you perform each movement mindfully and safely.

SHOULDER AND UPPER BODY RELAXATION TECHNIQUES

Shoulder tension can be a real burden, affecting your shoulders, overall posture, and well-being. Stress often manifests in the shoulders, causing them to tighten and restrict movement. When your shoulders are tense, it impacts your upper body mobility, making even simple tasks feel strenuous. This tension also disrupts your posture, leading to a cycle of discomfort and strain that can affect your daily life. Poor posture from slouched shoulders can even lead to headaches and neck pain, further complicating your physical health. To alleviate this tension, specific somatic exercises can work wonders.

One simple yet effective exercise is **Shoulder Rolls**:

1. Sit or stand with your back straight.
2. Calmly lift your shoulders up to your ears and then roll them back and down.
3. Repeat this motion several times to release built-up tension.

Arm Circles are another great option:

1. Extend your arms out to the sides and move them in small, controlled circles.
2. Slowly increase the size of the circles to enhance the stretch.
3. Shoulder blade squeezes are also beneficial.
4. Sit or stand with your back straight and squeeze your shoulder blades together (enough to hold a pencil between them).
5. Hold for a few seconds, and then release.

These exercises help to mobilize the shoulders, improve flexibility, and reduce tension.

In addition to these exercises, therapeutic techniques can further enhance shoulder relaxation. For example, a **Foam Roller** for your upper back and shoulders can relieve deep tissue.

1. Lie on your back with the foam roller and place it under your upper back.
2. Slowly roll back and forth.
3. Focus on areas that feel tight.

This technique helps to soften up knots and improve circulation.

Gentle Self-Massage is another effective method. Using your fingers, apply gentle pressure to tight spots in your shoulders and upper back. This can help to ease tension and relax your muscles.

Maintaining good posture and ergonomics is crucial for preventing shoulder tension. A proper desk setup can make a significant difference. Ensure your chair supports your lower back, and your computer is at eye level. This setup helps to keep your shoulders relaxed and your spine aligned. Ergonomic adjustments in your daily activities are also necessary. When lifting objects, use your legs rather than your back to avoid straining your shoulders. While sitting, keep your shoulders back and your feet flat on the floor. These minor adjustments can help to prevent shoulder tension and improve your overall posture.

RELEASING TENSION IN THE HIPS

Stress has a sneaky way of settling into our hips, often without us realizing it. Emotional stress, for instance, can cause our bodies to tense up, and the hips are no exception. They act like emotional sponges, soaking up stress and holding onto it, which can lead to tightness and discomfort. Prolonged sitting only makes things worse. When you sit for long periods of time, your hip flexors remain in a shortened position, leading to tightness and reduced mobility. This combination of emotional stress and physical inactivity can make your hips feel like they're made of stone.

To counteract this, specific somatic exercises can help release hip tension and improve flexibility.

Start with **Hip Flexor Stretches**:

1. Stand with one foot forward and the other back, bending your front knee while keeping your back leg straight.

2. Push your hips forward slowly until you feel a stretch in the front of your hip.
3. Hold it for a few seconds and switch sides.

Pigeon Pose is another excellent stretch:

1. Begin in a tabletop position.
2. Bring one knee forward and extend the other leg straight back.
3. Lower your chest toward the ground and relax into the stretch, feeling the release in your hips.

Seated Forward Bends can also be very effective:

1. Sit with your legs extended straight forward.
2. Slowly reach forward.
3. Aim to touch your toes while keeping your back straight.

This stretch is for the hamstrings and lower back, relieving the entire lower body.

Butterfly Stretches are great for opening the hips:

1. Sit while keeping the soles of your feet together, and your knees spread outward.
2. Gently push your knees toward the ground with your elbows while leaning forward slightly.

This stretch helps to ease tension and improve flexibility in the inner thighs and hips.

The benefits of these exercises are multifaceted. By releasing hip tension, you can significantly improve your overall mobility. Increased hip flexibility allows for a greater range of motion, making everyday activities like walking and sitting more comfortable. Reducing overall tension in the lower body also helps to alleviate pain and discomfort, contributing to a sense of ease and well-being. These improvements can make it easier to engage in other physical activities, enhancing your overall fitness and health.

Adding these practices into your daily routine is straightforward. Start with a morning mobility routine to wake up your hips and prepare them for the day ahead. This could include a few minutes of hip flexor stretches and Pigeon Pose. After long periods of sitting, take a break to perform seated forward bends and butterfly stretches. These movements can help to counteract the effects of prolonged sitting, keeping your hips flexible and relaxed. In the evening, wind down with gentle hip stretches to release any accumulated tension from the day. This practice can promote relaxation and improve sleep quality.

By making these exercises a regular part of your daily routine, you can keep your hips healthy, flexible, and pain-free. Consistency is key, so aim to practice these stretches daily, even if only for a few minutes. Your hips will thank you for it, and you'll enjoy the benefits of improved mobility and reduced tension throughout your lower body.

FULL-BODY TENSION RELEASE ROUTINE

Taking a holistic approach to releasing tension in your body can yield significant benefits for your overall well-being. When you focus on comprehensive stress reduction, you address isolated areas of discomfort and the interconnected web of tension that can spread throughout your body. This approach helps improve flexibility and mobility, allowing you to move more freely and comfortably. Enhanced body awareness is another key benefit. Regularly engaging in full-body routines makes you more tuned into the subtle signals your body sends you, enabling you to respond to stress and tension more effectively.

CHAPTER 3

A full-body tension release routine begins with gentle warm-up exercises. These exercises equip your muscles and joints for the movements to come, reducing the risk of injury. Start with simple activities like shaking out your hands and feet, rolling your shoulders, and gently twisting your torso. These movements increase blood flow and awaken your body, making it more receptive to deeper stretches and exercises. Once warmed up, transition to the main full-body stretches and movements. These can include a series of flowing movements that engage multiple muscle groups. For example, start with a standing forward bend to stretch your hamstrings and lower back, then move into a lunge to open your hips and stretch your legs.

After engaging in these dynamic movements, it's time to wind down with relaxation techniques. These exercises help to calm your nervous system and release any residual tension. Lie on your back with your legs up the wall, a restorative pose that encourages blood flow and relaxation. Practice deep breathing while in this position, inhaling fully through your nose and exhaling slowly through your mouth. This combination of physical relaxation and mindful breathing helps to fully release tension and prepare your body for rest.

Consistency is crucial for achieving long-term benefits from your full-body routine. Scheduling regular practice sessions ensures that you make time for this important self-care activity. Whether it's daily or several times a week, having a set schedule helps you stay committed. Tracking your progress and making adjustments as needed can also be highly motivating. Keep a journal to note how you feel before and after each session, and make any necessary tweaks to your routine based on your observations.

To make this routine accessible for everyone, consider offering modifications for different fitness levels. Beginner-friendly adaptations might include using props like pillows or straps to assist with stretches or performing movements at a slower pace. For advanced practitioners, deeper stretches and more challenging movements can be incorporated to increase the intensity. For example, beginners might perform a gentle lunge, while advanced practitioners could transition into a deeper warrior pose. These modifications ensure everyone can benefit from the routine, regardless of their starting point.

DAILY ROUTINE FOR MANAGING CHRONIC PAIN

Creating a structured routine can be a game-changer in managing chronic pain. Start your morning with neck stretches to gently wake up your muscles. Sit comfortably and perform side-to-side neck stretches, followed by forward and backward tilts, and finish with neck rotations. These exercises help release any tension accumulated overnight, setting a positive tone for the day.

As the day progresses, take a few moments around midday to focus on back movements. Whether you're at work or home, stand up and perform a series of pelvic tilts and cat-cow stretches. These movements are simple yet effective in relieving lower back tension, especially if you've been sitting for extended periods. Follow these with shoulder blade squeezes and thoracic spine rotations to address any upper back stiffness. These exercises keep your back flexible and reduce the risk of pain building up throughout the day.

In the evening, shift your focus to shoulder relaxation techniques. After a long day, your shoulders likely carry a significant amount of tension. Begin with shoulder rolls and arm circles to loosen up the muscles. Incorporate therapeutic techniques like using a foam roller for your upper back and shoulders or gentle self-massage. These methods can provide relief, promote relaxation, and prepare your body for a restful night.

CHAPTER 3

Consistency is key to effectively reducing chronic pain. Regular practice of somatic exercises brings long-term relief by gradually reducing the tension stored in your muscles. Daily routines help reinforce these benefits, making it easier to manage pain. The more consistent you are, the more your body will adapt, leading to sustained improvements over time.

Incorporating mindfulness practices can enhance the effectiveness of your routine. Start the day with a body scan, paying attention to any areas of tension and making a mental note to address them later. Use breath awareness throughout your exercises, inhaling deeply and exhaling slowly to promote relaxation. This approach helps you stay present and connected to your body, making the exercises more effective.

Adaptation is crucial for fitting these routines into your life. On busy days, shorten the exercises to a few minutes each, focusing on the most critical areas. On days when you have more time, add extra repetitions or variations to deepen the stretches. This flexibility ensures you can maintain your routine regardless of your schedule, making it a sustainable practice.

In summary, a structured daily routine that includes morning neck stretches, midday back movements and evening shoulder relaxation techniques can significantly improve one's ability to manage chronic pain. Consistency, mindfulness, and adaptability are key elements that make this routine effective and sustainable. Integrating these practices into one's daily life creates a foundation for long-term well-being and pain relief.

CHAPTER 4
BODY-FOCUSED HEALING FOR TRAUMA AND PTSD

GROUNDING TECHNIQUES FOR TRAUMA SURVIVORS

Grounding techniques are vital for trauma survivors for several reasons. When you've experienced trauma, your emotions can feel like a storm, unpredictable and overwhelming. Grounding helps to stabilize these emotions, providing a sense of control and calm. It also reduces dissociation, a common response to trauma where you might feel disconnected from your body or surroundings. By anchoring you in the present, grounding techniques enhance your awareness of the here and now, making it easier to navigate daily life without being pulled back into traumatic memories.

Physical Grounding Techniques are straightforward yet powerful. One effective method is stomping your feet on the ground:

- Stand up and firmly plant your feet on the floor.
- Lift one foot and stomp it back down with intention.
- Repeat with the other foot.

The physical sensation of your feet connecting with the ground can help you feel more present and anchored.

Another technique involves holding and squeezing a stress ball. The tactile sensation of the ball in your hand and the repetitive squeezing motion can bring your focus back to the present moment. Walking barefoot on surfaces like grass, dirt, or sand is another excellent grounding exercise. The textures and temperatures you feel underfoot can help you reconnect with your body and the world around you.

Sensory Grounding Exercises engage your senses to keep you connected to your environment:

- Start by describing objects in the room around you. Choose an item and focus on its color, shape, texture, and any other details you can see. Saying these observations out loud can enhance the grounding effect.
- Focusing on different textures is another effective method. Rub your hands over various surfaces, such as a soft blanket, a wooden table, or a smooth stone. Pay attention to how each texture feels under your fingers.
- Engaging with soothing scents can also be grounding. Use essential oils (lavender or chamomile), or light a scented candle. Inhale deeply and focus on the aroma, allowing it to center your thoughts.

Visualization Grounding Techniques can be incredibly calming. One effective method is imagining roots growing from your feet into the ground:

- Sit or stand comfortably and close your eyes.
- Visualize strong roots extending from your feet, going deep into the earth.

- Feel the stability and support these roots provide, anchoring you firmly in the present moment.

Another visualization involves imagining a safe, stable place. Close your eyes and picture a location where you feel completely secure and at peace. It could be a real place you've visited or a purely imaginary one. Focus on the details—the sounds, smells, and sights of this place. Allow the sense of safety to envelop you, grounding you in the here and now.

Incorporating these grounding techniques into your routine can make a significant difference in managing trauma and PTSD symptoms. Whether you're stomping your feet, describing objects in the room, or visualizing roots growing from your feet, these practices help stabilize your emotions, reduce dissociation, and enhance your present-moment awareness. They offer a practical, accessible way to navigate the challenges of trauma and reclaim a sense of control and peace in your life.

SOMATIC EXERCISES FOR EMOTIONAL RELEASE

Releasing stored emotions is vital for trauma survivors. When emotions are held in, they can build up over time, creating a pressure cooker situation that can hinder both your mental and physical well-being. This buildup can lead to heightened anxiety, depression, and even physical conditions like headaches and muscle tension. Allowing these emotions to surface and be expressed can promote psychological healing, helping you process past experiences and move forward with a lighter, clearer mind.

Movement-Based Release Exercises are an excellent way to tap into these stored emotions and let them flow. One effective method is shaking exercises:

- Stand with your feet shoulder-width apart.

- Shake your entire body.
- Start gently and gradually increase the intensity.
- Shake your arms, legs, and torso, letting every part of your body move freely.

This activity helps dislodge stuck energy and emotions, allowing them to be released.

Another powerful exercise is **Dancing Freely** to music:

- Choose a song that resonates with you and let your body move however it wants.
- There are no rules or specific steps to follow—just let the music guide you.

This form of expression can be incredibly liberating and joyful.

Combining stretching with **Deep Breaths** is another effective technique:

- Start with a gentle stretch, such as reaching your arms overhead and elongating your spine.
- As you stretch, take a deep breath in through your nose, filling your lungs completely.
- Hold your breath for a few seconds and exhale slowly through your mouth, releasing any tension.
- Repeat this process with different stretches, focusing on areas where you feel tight or tense.

The mix of physical movement and controlled breathing can help release stored emotions and promote a sense of relaxation.

Vocal Release Techniques can also be incredibly therapeutic. Humming is a simple yet effective way to release emotion:

- Find a comfortable place to sit and close your eyes.
- Take a deep breath in and hum as you exhale.
- Feel the vibrations in your chest and throat, allowing the sound to resonate throughout your body.

Chanting is another powerful method:

- Choose a word or phrase that feels meaningful to you, such as "peace" or "calm."
- Repeat the word or phrase out loud, letting the sound fill the space around you.

Allowing spontaneous vocal expressions can also be liberating. Find a private space where you feel safe and let any sounds that come to you emerge. This could be yelling, crying, laughing, or any other vocal expression that feels right.

Creative activities like writing and drawing can also aid in emotional release. Journaling about your emotions provides a safe space to explore and process your feelings. Set aside time each day to write freely about whatever comes to mind. Don't worry about grammar or structure—just let your thoughts flow onto the paper. Drawing or painting your feelings is another expressive outlet. Gather some art supplies and let your emotions guide your hand. You might create abstract shapes, detailed images, or something in between. The act of creating can help externalize your emotions, making them easier to understand and release.

Incorporating these somatic exercises for emotional release into your routine can help you manage the emotional weight of trauma. Movement, vocal expression, and creative activities provide various outlets for emotions, allowing you to process and release them in a healthy, constructive way. Whether you're shaking off tension, dancing to your favorite song, or journaling about your day, these practices offer valuable tools for emotional healing and well-being.

TRAUMA-INFORMED BREATHWORK PRACTICES

Trauma-informed breathwork is a specialized approach that acknowledges the individual needs and triggers of trauma survivors. It's not just about breathing exercises; it's about constructing a safe, supportive environment where you can reconnect with your body at your own pace. Sensitivity to trauma triggers is paramount. Some breathing techniques might inadvertently bring up distressing memories or emotions, so a gradual approach to breath awareness is crucial. Instead of diving straight into deep breathing exercises, you start slowly, observing your natural breath without trying to change it. This helps you become comfortable with feeling your breath and builds a foundation for more advanced practices.

Begin with simple exercises to develop **Initial Breath Awareness**:

- Sit or lie down in a comfortable position.
- Close your eyes if you feel safe doing so.
- Start by observing your natural breath without altering it.
- Take note of the air entering and leaving your nostrils.
- Take note of the rise and fall of your stomach.
- This simple act of observation can be profoundly grounding.
- Next, place your hands on your abdomen.
- As you inhale, feel your abdomen rise.
- As you exhale, feel it fall.

This tactile feedback helps you connect more deeply with your breath and can be very soothing.

Once you're comfortable with basic breath awareness, you can move on to calming breath techniques designed to help regulate your nervous system.

The **4-7-8 Breathing** technique:

- Inhale gradually through your nose for four seconds.
- Hold your breath for seven seconds.
- Fully exhale through your mouth for eight seconds.

This helps activate the parasympathetic nervous system for relaxation and reduces stress.

Another effective technique is **Coherent Breathing**:

- Inhale for five seconds.
- Exhale for five seconds.

This balanced breathing pattern helps create a sense of calm and stability.

For those further along in their trauma recovery, advanced **Trauma-Informed Breathwork Techniques** can offer deeper benefits. Box breathing is one such technique:

- It involves inhaling for a count of four seconds.
- Hold your breath for four seconds.
- Exhale for four seconds.
- Hold again for four seconds.

This method calms the mind and improves focus and emotional resilience.

Alternate Nostril Breathing is another powerful practice:

- Sit comfortably.
- Use your thumb to close your right nostril.
- Inhale through your left nostril.
- Close your left nostril with your finger, release your thumb, and exhale through your right nostril.
- Inhale through the right nostril, close it with your thumb, release your finger, and exhale through the left nostril.

Alternate nostril breathing balances the brain's hemispheres, promotes mental clarity, and reduces stress.

Incorporating trauma-informed breathwork into your routine can make a significant difference in managing trauma-related symptoms. These practices are designed to be gentle and supportive, helping you reconnect with your body in a safe and empowering way. Remember, the key is to go at your own pace, listen to your body, and choose the techniques that resonate with you. As you become more comfortable with these exercises, you'll find that breathwork can be a powerful tool for healing and emotional regulation.

INCORPORATING BREATHWORK FOR TRAUMA RECOVERY

Breathwork is a powerful tool for trauma recovery, offering both physiological and psychological benefits. When you engage in controlled breathing, you influence your body's autonomic nervous system. This can help switch off the "fight or flight" response, which is often overactive in trauma survivors. Physiologically, breathwork can lower your heart rate, reduce blood pressure, and lower levels of cortisol. Psychologically, controlled breathing promotes a sense of calm and can improve emotional regulation. It allows you to create a buffer between your immediate reactions and more measured responses, helping you manage anxiety and stress more effectively.

Let's delve into some specific breathwork techniques that support trauma recovery.

Diaphragmatic Breathing (Belly Breathing) is a simple yet effective technique:

- Find a comfortable position to sit or lie down.
- Place one hand on your chest and the other on your stomach.
- Breathe in through your nose and allow your stomach to rise while keeping your chest relatively still.
- Exhale calmly through your mouth and feel your stomach fall.

This method engages your diaphragm and promotes relaxation.

Box Breathing is another fantastic technique for calming the nervous system:

- Sit comfortably and close your eyes if you feel safe doing so.
- Inhale through your nose for four seconds.
- Hold your breath for four seconds.
- Exhale calmly through your mouth for four seconds.
- Finally, hold your breath again for four seconds.

This creates a rhythmic pattern that can help calm your emotions and balance.

Alternate Nostril Breathing is particularly effective for balancing the hemispheres of your brain and promoting mental clarity:

- Sit in a comfortable position and use your thumb to close off your right nostril.
- Inhale through your left nostril.
- Close your left nostril with your finger, release your thumb, and exhale through your right nostril.
- Inhale through the right nostril, close it with your thumb again and release your finger to exhale through the left nostril.

This technique can help you feel more centered and focused.

Integrating breathwork with other somatic practices can enhance its effectiveness. Combining breathwork with movement, for example, can deepen the impact. Try incorporating diaphragmatic breathing into your stretching routines. As you stretch, inhale deeply and exhale slowly, allowing your breath to guide your movement. This combination can help release physical tension and promote a deeper sense of relaxation.

Adding breathwork into your daily routine can make it easier to manage trauma-related symptoms.

Here's a step-by-step guide for a **Breathwork Routine** that you can follow to incorporate these practices into your daily life:

- Begin your morning with five minutes of diaphragmatic breathing. Sit or lie down, put one hand on your chest and the other on your abdomen, and breathe deeply.
- For anxiety relief during the day, practice box breathing for three to five minutes whenever you feel overwhelmed.
- In the evening, spend five minutes on alternate nostril breathing. Find a quiet space, sit comfortably, and follow the technique as described.

CHAPTER 4

By incorporating these breathwork techniques into your daily routine and combining them with other somatic practices, you can create a holistic approach to trauma recovery. This integrated practice can help you manage symptoms more effectively and promote long-term healing and well-being.

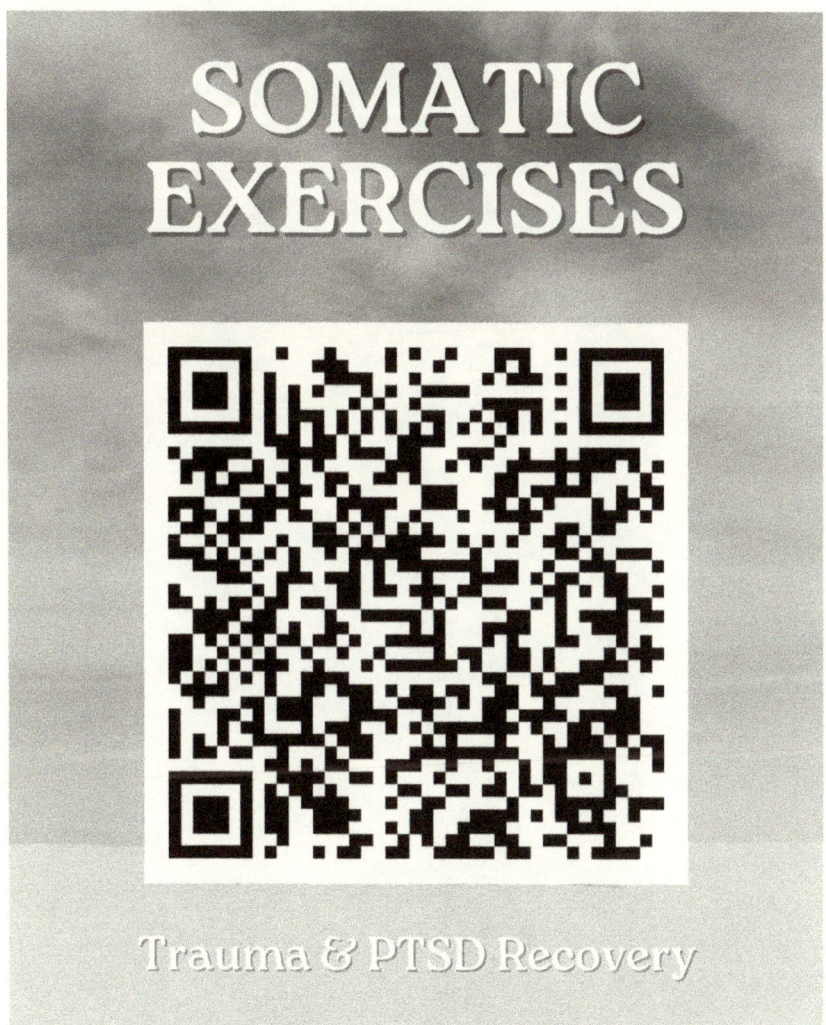

CHAPTER 5
CALMING THE NERVOUS SYSTEM FOR ANXIETY RELIEF

BREATHWORK FOR ANXIETY: TECHNIQUES TO CALM THE MIND AND BALANCE THE BODY

The biological impact of breath on anxiety is profound. When you feel anxious, your breathing tends to become shallow and rapid, signaling your body that danger is near. This rapid breathing, or hyperventilation, can lead to an imbalance of oxygen and carbon dioxide in your blood, exacerbating feelings of panic and discomfort. Controlled breathing helps restore balance, ensuring your body receives oxygen while maintaining a calm and steady heart rate. This physiological shift can significantly reduce anxiety symptoms and promote a sense of calm.

Breathwork affects the parasympathetic nervous system by stimulating the vagus nerve, which stretches from the brain to the abdomen and helps regulate various bodily functions, including heart rate and digestion. When you engage in controlled breathing, you activate this nerve, prompting the parasympathetic system to kick in. This activation slows down your heart rate, lowers blood pressure, and creates a state of relaxation. In essence, breathwork acts as a natural tranquilizer for your nervous system.

Let's explore some basic calming breath techniques you can practice today. **Deep Belly Breathing (diaphragmatic breathing)** is a simple yet effective method:

1. Sit or lie down in a comfy position.
2. Place one hand on your chest and the other on your stomach.
3. Inhale deeply through your nose, raising your abdomen (keeping your chest as still as you can).
4. Exhale slowly through your mouth while you feel your stomach fall.
5. Repeat this process for several minutes.
6. Focus on the rise and fall of your stomach.

Another effective technique is **4-4-4-4 Box Breathing**:

1. Sit comfortably and close your eyes if you feel safe doing so.
2. Inhale through your nose for four seconds.
3. Hold your breath for four seconds.
4. Exhale calmly through your mouth for four seconds.
5. Hold your breath for another four seconds before starting the cycle again.

This method creates a rhythmic pattern that can help regulate your emotions and bring a feeling of balance.

Equal Breathing (Sama Vritti) is another excellent option:

1. Sit comfortably and close your eyes.
2. Inhale through your nose for four seconds.
3. Exhale through your nose for four seconds.

4. The goal is to make your inhales and exhales equal in length, creating a balanced and calming effect on your nervous system.

Advanced techniques can offer deeper benefits for those with some experience in breathwork. **Alternate Nostril Breathing (Nadi Shodhana)** is a powerful practice:

1. Sit comfortably.
2. Use your thumb to close your right nostril.
3. Inhale through your left nostril.
4. Close your left nostril with your finger, release your thumb, and exhale through your right nostril.
5. Inhale through your right nostril, close it with your thumb, and release your finger to exhale through the left nostril.

This technique balances the brain's hemispheres, promoting mental clarity and reducing stress.

Resonance Breathing (5-5 pattern) helps create a sense of calm and stability:

1. Inhale for five seconds.
2. Exhale for five seconds.

Another advanced technique is **2:1 Breathing**, where your exhalation is twice as long as your inhalation. For example:

1. Inhale for three seconds.
2. Exhale for six seconds.

This method promotes relaxation by extending the exhalation phase, which is associated with activating the parasympathetic nervous system.

Integrating breathwork into your daily life can make it easier to manage anxiety:

1. Start your day with a morning breathwork routine. Spend a few minutes practicing deep belly breathing to set a calm tone for the day.
2. During stressful situations, use box breathing to center yourself and reduce anxiety.
3. In the evening, wind down with equal breathing or alternate nostril breathing to prepare your body and mind for restful sleep.

Adding breathwork to your daily routine can create a powerful foundation for managing anxiety. These techniques offer practical, accessible tools you can use anytime, anywhere. By making breathwork a regular part of your life, you can cultivate a sense of calm and resilience that supports your overall well-being.

SOMATIC PRACTICES FOR MANAGING PANIC ATTACKS

Panic attacks can be terrifying and make you feel like you are out of control. They involve both physiological and psychological responses that can be overwhelming. When you experience a panic attack, your body activates the fight-or-flight response, a survival mechanism designed to protect you from danger. This response floods your body with adrenaline, causing your heart rate to spike, your breathing to become rapid, and your muscles to tense. These physical symptoms can be alarming, making you feel as though something terrible is happening. Psychologically, panic attacks often include intense fear, a sense of impending doom, and a feeling of detachment from reality.

CHAPTER 5

Common triggers for panic attacks vary from person to person. They can include stressful situations, specific phobias, or even seemingly minor events that remind you of past trauma. Symptoms often appear suddenly and can include sweating, shaking, chest pain, dizziness, and a feeling of choking. These symptoms can be debilitating, disrupting your ability to function in daily life.

Somatic practices can be highly effective in managing and reducing the intensity of panic attacks. One helpful technique is the **5-4-3-2-1 Grounding** exercise. This method helps anchor you in the present moment by engaging your senses:

1. Start by identifying five things you can see around you.
2. Next, focus on four things you can touch.
3. Then, listen for three different sounds.
4. Identify two things you can smell.
5. Find one thing you can taste.

This exercise takes your focus away from the panic and onto your immediate environment, helping to calm your mind and body.

Slow, **Deep Breathing** is another powerful tool for managing panic attacks. When you feel a panic attack coming on, find a quiet space if possible:

1. Sit down, close your eyes, and take a deep breath through your nose, allowing your abdomen to expand.
2. Hold your breath for a few seconds.
3. Exhale slowly through your mouth.
4. Repeat this process several times.
5. Focus on the feeling of your breath moving in and out of your body.
6. This practice can help slow your heart rate and reduce the physical symptoms of panic.

Tension and Release Exercises can also provide relief. These practices involve tensing and relaxing different muscle groups to release built-up tension:

1. Start by sitting or lying down comfortably.
2. Tense the muscles in your feet.
3. Hold for a few seconds and release.
4. Move your focus up to your calves, thighs, stomach, chest, and arms.
5. End with your face.

This systematic approach helps to release tension and creates a sense of relaxation throughout your body.

Preparation and practice are key to ensuring these techniques are effective during a panic attack. It's essential to practice these exercises regularly in low-stress situations. This helps you become familiar with the techniques and makes it easier to use them when you need them most. Building a toolkit of techniques ensures you have multiple strategies to rely on, increasing your chances of finding relief.

Here's a step-by-step guide for managing a panic attack. When you feel a panic attack starting, begin with immediate response techniques like slow, deep breathing to calm your body. Next, use mid-attack grounding exercises such as the 5-4-3-2-1 technique to shift your focus away from the panic. After the attack subsides, engage in post-attack recovery methods such as tension and release exercises to help your body return to a state of relaxation. By following this structured routine, you can manage the intensity of panic attacks and reduce their impact on your life.

CHAPTER 5

DAILY ANXIETY-REDUCING ROUTINES

Establishing consistent daily routines can be a game-changer in managing anxiety. When you create structure and predictability in your day, it helps to reduce overall anxiety levels. Knowing what to expect and when can make you feel more in control, easing the mental burden of constant decision-making. Decision fatigue is real and can exacerbate feelings of anxiety. By having set routines, you minimize the number of choices you need to make each day, saving your mental energy for other important tasks. This structure can make your day flow more smoothly, providing a sense of stability and calm.

Morning mindfulness practices can set the tone for a balanced day. Begin your day with a few minutes of quiet reflection or meditation. Find a comfortable spot, close your eyes, and focus on the present moment. This practice can help you start your day with a clear mind and a calm heart. Another effective morning routine is journaling. Spend a few minutes writing down your thoughts, goals, or things you're grateful for. This can help you organize your mind and set positive intentions for the day ahead. Incorporating these practices into your daily morning routine can create a foundation of tranquility that carries you through the day.

Midday movement breaks are essential for reducing anxiety levels. Taking short breaks to move your body can help interrupt the cycle of stress and tension. Simple activities like stretching, walking around the block, or even a quick dance session can make a significant difference. Movement releases endorphins, which are your body's natural stress relievers and help break up the day's monotony. If you work in an office, set an alarm to remind yourself to stretch every hour. Even a few minutes of movement can refresh your mind and reduce physical tension.

Evening relaxation routines are crucial for winding down and preparing for restful sleep. Create a calming ritual that signals your body that it's time to relax. This could be activities like reading a book, taking a long bath, or engaging in gentle yoga. Try to avoid screens and bright lights at least an hour before bed, as these can hinder your body's natural sleep signals. Instead, opt for calming activities that promote relaxation. Listening to soothing music or practicing gratitude can also be effective. By establishing a consistent evening routine, you help your body transition smoothly from the day's activities to a state of rest.

Physical activity plays a significant role in anxiety reduction. Regular exercise helps regulate your stress response and can quickly alleviate anxiety. Incorporate gentle stretching routines into your daily life to keep your muscles relaxed and flexible. Simple stretches like reaching for your toes, rolling your shoulders, or twisting your torso can make a big difference. Walking is another fantastic option. A brisk walk and fresh air can clear your mind and improve your mood. If you prefer more structured exercise, consider light activities like yoga or tai chi. These practices combine movement with mindfulness, offering a double benefit for reducing anxiety.

Creating and maintaining these routines can be challenging, but practical tips can make it easier. Setting reminders and alarms on your smartphone can help you stay on track. Use habit-tracking apps to monitor your goals and keep you motivated. Finding accountability partners can also be beneficial. Share your goals with friends with similar interests. Having someone to check in with can encourage you to stick with your routines.

VISUALIZATION TECHNIQUES TO EASE ANXIETY

Visualization is an effective tool for easing anxiety by creating calming mental images. It taps into the mind's incredible ability to

CHAPTER 5

influence emotions. When you visualize a serene scene or a comforting image, your brain often responds as if you are actually experiencing it. This can significantly reduce anxiety and promote a sense of calm. Visualization works because your brain cannot easily distinguish between real and imagined experiences. By harnessing this power, you can create a mental sanctuary that helps you navigate stressful moments more effectively.

One of the key benefits of visualization for anxiety relief is its ability to move focus away from anxious thoughts. When anxiety strikes, your mind can become a whirlwind of worries and fears. Visualization provides a mental escape, a way to step outside the storm and find peace. It can also help you build emotional resilience, giving you a mental toolkit to draw upon in challenging times. Regular practice can improve your overall mental well-being, making it easier to manage anxiety in the long term.

Let's start with some basic visualization exercises. **Safe Place Visualization** is a great way to begin:

1. Find a quiet space to sit or lie down comfortably.
2. Close your eyes and imagine a place where you feel completely safe and at ease.
3. It could be a real location, like a favorite beach, a cozy room, or an entirely imagined place.
4. Focus on the details: the colors, sounds, and textures.
5. Picture yourself there, feeling the safety and comfort of this place.
6. Spend a few minutes in this mental sanctuary, allowing it to soothe your mind and body.

Guided Imagery of a peaceful scene is another effective technique:

1. Imagine a serene landscape, such as a tranquil forest or a calm ocean.

2. Visualize yourself walking through this scene, noticing the sights, sounds, and smells around you.
3. Feel the ground beneath your feet, hear the birds sing, and take a deep breath of fresh air.

This exercise helps to transport your mind to a place of peace, reducing anxiety and promoting relaxation.

Visualizing a protective bubble can also be very calming. Sit comfortably and close your eyes. Imagine a warm, glowing bubble surrounding you. This bubble is impenetrable, keeping out any negative thoughts or stressors. Picture it as a shield that protects you from anxiety, allowing only positive, calming energy to enter. Spend a few minutes in this protective bubble, feeling safe and secure.

More advanced practices can provide deeper benefits for those comfortable with basic visualizations. Future self-visualization involves imagining yourself in the future, having overcome current challenges, and feeling confident and happy. Picture your future self in a specific scenario, such as giving a successful presentation or enjoying a peaceful moment. Focus on the emotions associated with this future success. This exercise can boost your confidence and reduce anxiety by reinforcing positive outcomes.

Healing Light Visualization is another advanced technique:

1. Sit or lie down and close your eyes.
2. Imagine a warm, radiant light above you.
3. Visualize this light slowly descending, entering the top of your head, and filling your entire body.
4. As the light moves through you, it heals and soothes every part it touches, dissolving any tension or anxiety.
5. Feel this healing light enveloping you, bringing a profound sense of peace and relaxation.

CHAPTER 5

To enhance the effectiveness of visualization exercises, engage all five senses. When imagining a scene, think about what you can see, hear, smell, touch, and taste. This multisensory approach makes the visualization more vivid and immersive. Practicing regularly can also yield better results. Set aside a few minutes each day for visualization, making it a consistent part of your routine. Combining visualization with breathwork can amplify the calming effects. For example, practice deep belly breathing while visualizing a peaceful scene, synchronizing your breath with the imagery.

By incorporating visualization strategies into your daily life, you can create a mental refuge that helps to manage and reduce anxiety. These exercises offer a simple but powerful way to harness the mind's ability to influence emotions, providing a valuable tool for emotional regulation and well-being.

CHAPTER 6
OVERCOMING DEPRESSION AND LOW ENERGY

ENERGIZING MORNING ROUTINES

Starting your day with an energizing routine can set a positive tone for the day. You lay the groundwork for a more productive and joyful day when you wake up and take part in activities that boost your energy and mood. Consistency in these routines is key. When you make them a daily habit, you create a rhythm that your body and mind can rely on, which helps reduce decision fatigue and sets a proactive mindset.

One of the first things you can do to boost your energy in the morning is gentle stretching. As soon as you wake up, take a few moments to stretch your body. Reach your arms overhead, stretch your legs, and gently twist your torso. These movements help wake up your muscles and increase blood flow, making you feel more alert and ready to face the day. Light aerobic movements, such as marching in place or doing a few jumping jacks, can further invigorate your body. These activities elevate your heart rate and stimulate the release of endorphins, which are natural mood enhancers.

Another powerful exercise to include in your morning routine is the **Sun Salutation** sequence, a series of yoga poses designed to energize the body and mind:

1. Start by standing tall with your feet together and hands in prayer position at your chest.
2. Inhale deeply, raise your arms overhead and look up.
3. Exhale as you bend forward, reaching for your toes.
4. Inhale again as you lift halfway up, flattening your back.
5. Exhale and step back into a plank position, then lower your body to the floor.
6. Inhale as you lift your chest into a gentle backbend, and exhale as you push back into a downward-facing dog pose.
7. Finally, walk your feet forward, inhale as you lift halfway, exhale as you fold forward, and inhale as you rise back up to standing.

This sequence stretches and strengthens your muscles and synchronizes your breath with movement, leaving you feeling revitalized.

Incorporating mindfulness techniques into your morning routine can enhance its effectiveness. Start with a morning gratitude practice. Before getting out of bed, take a few moments to think about three things you're grateful for. This small act can flip your mindset from a place of scarcity to one of abundance.

Mindful breathing exercises are another excellent addition. Sit comfortably and take a couple deep breaths. Focus on the feeling of the air entering and leaving your body. This practice helps center your mind and prepare you for the day ahead. Setting positive intentions for the day can also be powerful. Take a moment to think about what you want to achieve or how you want to feel. This intention-setting can guide your actions and keep you focused on what truly matters.

Creating a personalized morning routine ensures that it fits your unique needs and preferences. Choose exercises that feel invigorating to you. If you enjoy yoga, incorporate poses that stretch and energize your body. If dancing lifts your spirits, start your day with a few minutes of your favorite tunes. Adjust the duration of your routine based on your time availability. Even a five-minute routine can make a significant difference. Keeping a morning routine journal can help you track your progress and notice the benefits over time. Note how you feel before and after your routine, and make adjustments as needed. This reflection can motivate you to stay consistent and make your mornings a time of renewal and positivity.

MOVEMENT PRACTICES TO LIFT MOOD

Physical movement can profoundly impact your mood and mental health. When you take part in physical activity, your body releases endorphins, often called "feel-good" hormones. These natural chemicals communicate with receptors in your brain, reducing your perception of pain and creating positive feelings. Additionally, movement helps reduce levels of stress hormones like cortisol, which can hurt your emotional well-being if left unchecked. Improved blood circulation is another significant benefit. When your blood flows more freely, it delivers extra oxygen and nutrients to your cells, boosting energy levels and mental clarity. This combination of biochemical and physiological changes can nurture a more balanced emotional state, making it easier to cope with life's challenges.

Dance therapy exercises are particularly effective for lifting your mood. Find a space where you can move freely and put on some music that makes you want to dance. Start with simple movements, like swaying your hips or tapping your feet. As you get more comfortable, let your body move more freely. There's no right or wrong way to dance in this context—it's all about expressing yourself and releasing pent-up energy. Tai Chi, a form of martial arts that focuses on slow, deliberate movements, is another excellent practice. These movements promote relaxation and mental focus, helping to alleviate symptoms of depression and anxiety. Rhythmic walking or jogging can also be incredibly uplifting. Find a path in your neighborhood or a nearby park and set a steady pace. The repetitive motion can be meditative, providing both physical exercise and mental relief.

Creative movement exercises offer another way to enhance your mood through physical activity. Free-form dancing is a fantastic option. Unlike dance therapy, which might have some structure, free-form dancing is all about letting your body move in whatever way feels right. Close your eyes if it helps you feel less self-conscious, and just move to the music. Movement improvisation can also be liberating. This involves creating spontaneous movements in response to your environment or internal feelings. For example, you might mimic the flow of a river with your arms or the swaying of trees in the wind. Incorporating music into these movements can further amplify their mood-lifting effects. Choose songs that resonate with you emotionally, whether they're upbeat and energetic or slow and soothing.

To make movement enjoyable, find ways to inject joy into the experience. Choose your favorite music or playlists to accompany your activities. Music has a powerful influence on mood and can make physical exercise feel less like a chore and more like a celebration. Moving in natural or outdoor settings can also enhance the experience. Fresh air, sunlight, and natural scenery can uplift your spirits and provide a change of environment that invigorates both body and mind. Practicing with a partner or group can add a social element that makes movement more enjoyable. Whether it's a dance class, a Tai Chi group, or a walking club, sharing the experience with others can provide motivation and make the activity more fun.

Incorporating these movement practices into your routine can create a reliable way to lift your mood and improve your mental health. The key is to find what resonates with you and make it a regular part of your life. When you enjoy the activities you engage in, you're more likely to stick with them, reaping the emotional and physical benefits they offer. Whether you're dancing in your living room, practicing Tai Chi in the park, or going for a rhythmic jog, these practices can help you release trauma, stress, and emotional tension stored in your body.

BREATHWORK TO COMBAT FATIGUE

Feeling fatigued can be more than just a nuisance; it can make even simple tasks feel insurmountable. Breathwork can be a powerful tool in combating this fatigue, helping you feel more energized and alert. When you engage in specific breathwork practices, you oxygenate your body more effectively. This means your blood carries more oxygen to your cells, boosting energy levels and overall vitality. Additionally, breathwork activates the parasympathetic nervous system, which promotes relaxation and helps counteract the stress that often contributes to fatigue. Improved mental clarity is another significant benefit. When your brain receives ample oxygen, it functions more efficiently, enhancing focus and sharpness.

One of the most energizing breathwork techniques is **Bellows Breath (Bhastrika)**. To perform this exercise:

1. Sit comfortably with your spine straight.
2. Inhale deeply through your nose, then do a hard exhale

through your nose, using your diaphragm to push the air out.
3. The breaths should be rapid and forceful, like the bellows of a blacksmith's forge.
4. Start with 10 breaths, then rest and breathe normally.
5. Gradually increase the number of breaths as you become more comfortable with the technique.

Bellows Breath stimulates your entire body, increasing oxygen flow and invigorating your mind.

Another effective technique is the **Breath of Joy**:

1. Stand with your feet hip-width apart and your knees slightly bent.
2. Inhale through your nose as you lift your arms in front of you.
3. With a second, sharper inhale, swing your arms out to the sides.
4. Finally, take a third, even sharper inhale as you lift your arms overhead.
5. Exhale through your mouth with a "ha" sound as you bend forward, letting your arms swing down and back.
6. Repeat this sequence several times.

The rhythmic, dynamic movement combined with deep breathing can increase energy and lift your mood.

Kapalabhati, or Skull Shining Breath, is another powerful breathwork practice. Sit comfortably with your spine straight. Take a deep breath in, then exhale with force through your nose by contracting your abdominal muscles. The inhalation should be passive, allowing your lungs to fill naturally. Focus on the forceful exhalation, repeating this process for 20-30 breaths. This technique increases oxygenation and helps clear your mind, making it an excellent practice for combating fatigue and enhancing mental clarity.

The **4-2-6-2 Breathing** pattern is highly effective for improving focus and mental sharpness:

1. Sit comfortably.
2. Inhale fully through your nose for four seconds.
3. Hold your breath for two seconds.
4. Exhale calmly through your mouth for a count of six, then hold your breath again for two seconds.
5. Repeat this cycle several times.

This pattern helps regulate your breathing, calm your mind, and sharpen your focus.

Single-Nostril Breathing is another technique that can enhance mental clarity:

1. Sit comfortably.
2. Use your thumb to close your right nostril.
3. Inhale through your left nostril.
4. Close your left nostril with your finger, release your thumb, and exhale through your right nostril.
5. Inhale through the right nostril, close it with your thumb, release your finger, and exhale through the left nostril.

This practice balances the hemispheres of your brain, promoting mental clarity and focus.

Incorporating breathwork into your daily life is straightforward and can be done at various times. Practice Bellows Breath or Breath of Joy for a few minutes for a mid-morning energy boost. These techniques can invigorate you when you start to feel sluggish. When fatigue often hits in the afternoon, try Kapalabhati or the 4-2-

6-2 breathing pattern to rejuvenate your energy levels and enhance focus. Before a meeting or any situation requiring mental sharpness, single-nostril breathing can help clear your mind and improve concentration.

These breathwork practices can be seamlessly integrated into your daily routine, providing a reliable and effective way to fight fatigue and enhance mental clarity. Whether you need a quick energy boost or a way to sharpen your focus, breathwork offers practical tools to help you feel more vibrant and alert.

AFTERNOON PICK-ME-UP EXERCISES

It's common to experience a dip in energy levels during the afternoon. This slump is often due to our natural circadian rhythms, which create a period of low alertness in the mid-afternoon. Your body's internal clock signals a downturn in energy, making it extra difficult to stay focused and productive. Diet and hydration also play crucial roles. Consuming heavy meals or not drinking enough water can exacerbate this fatigue. However, somatic exercises can help re-energize your body and mind, making the rest of your day more manageable.

One effective way to combat this slump is through quick stretching routines. Stand up, stretch your arms overhead, and slowly bend forward to touch your toes. This movement helps to release tension in your back and shoulders. Follow this with a gentle side stretch, reaching one arm over your head while bending to the opposite side. Repeat on the other side to balance out the stretch. These simple movements can increase blood flow and release built-up tension, making you more alert.

Energizing breathwork can also provide a much-needed boost. Try taking a few minutes to practice deep, **Diaphragmatic Breathing**:

CHAPTER 6

1. Sit comfortably.
2. Place one hand on your chest and the other on your stomach.
3. Inhale fully through your nose, feeling your stomach rise, then exhale slowly through your mouth.

This technique helps give your body oxygen and calm your mind, reducing fatigue.

Simple movement breaks can make a significant difference. Stand up and march in place for a minute or two. Swing your arms and lift your knees up to get your blood flowing. A short walk around your office or home can also be invigorating. These brief bursts of activity can break the monotony and revitalize your energy levels.

Hydration and nutrition are equally important. Drinking water or herbal teas can help keep you hydrated and alert. Dehydration is a common cause of fatigue, so make it a habit to sip water throughout the day. Herbal teas like peppermint or ginger are refreshing and provide a gentle energy boost. Eating energy-boosting snacks can also help. Opt for snacks that combine protein, healthy fats, and complex carbohydrates, such as nuts and a piece of fruit. These foods provide sustained energy without causing a sugar crash.

For an effective afternoon pick-me-up routine, start with a midday stretch sequence. Stand up and perform a series of stretches, including overhead reaches, forward bends, and side stretches. Next, practice a few minutes of energizing breathwork, focusing on deep, diaphragmatic breaths. Follow this with a simple movement break, such as marching in place or taking a short walk. Finally, ensure you stay hydrated by drinking a glass of water or herbal tea and enjoying a healthy snack to stabilize your energy levels.

Implementing this routine can help you navigate the afternoon slump more easily and vitality. Combining somatic exercises with proper hydration and nutrition allows you to maintain energy levels and stay productive throughout the day. Remember, small, consistent actions can lead to impactful improvements in your overall well-being.

CHAPTER 7
STRESS AND BURNOUT RECOVERY THROUGH MIND-BODY TECHNIQUES

INSTANT STRESS RELIEF TECHNIQUES

When stress hits suddenly, having quick relief techniques at your disposal is essential. These methods can help lower stress hormones like cortisol, preventing the situation from spiraling out of control. Imagine you're in a heated meeting at work, and you can feel the stress starting to build. Your heart races, your palms sweat, and your thoughts become jumbled. In moments like these, instant stress relief techniques can be a lifesaver. They help you regain control, enhance emotional regulation, and keep you calm in the face of a crisis.

Breath-based techniques are some of the most effective quick fixes for stress. One of the simplest and most accessible is **4-4-4-4 Box Breathing**. To practice this:

1. Sit comfortably and close your eyes if you can.
2. Inhale through your nose (four seconds).
3. Hold your breath (four seconds).

4. Exhale through your mouth (four seconds).
5. Hold again (four seconds).

This rhythmic breathing pattern helps calm your nervous system and brings your focus back to the present moment.

Another effective method is **5-5-5 Breathing**:

1. Inhale for five seconds.
2. Hold for five seconds.
3. Exhale for five seconds.

This technique is particularly useful for quickly reducing stress and anxiety.

The **Sighing Breath** is another great tool:

1. Take a deep inhale through your nose.
2. Hold for a moment.
3. Exhale audibly through your mouth, making a sighing sound.

This releases tension and signals to your body that it's safe to relax.

Somatic movements can be incredibly beneficial for those moments when you need a physical release. **Shoulder Shrug Exercises** are an easy way to help relieve tension:

1. Simply lift your shoulders up towards your ears and then let them drop back down.
2. Repeat this several times, feeling the tension melt away.
3. Palm presses can also provide instant relief.
4. Press your palms together in front of your chest, applying gentle pressure.
5. Hold for a few seconds before releasing.

CHAPTER 7

This action helps center your mind and body.

Neck Rolls are another effective technique:

- Gently roll your head in a circle motion.
- First in one direction and then the other.

This will help release tension in your neck and shoulders.

Sensory techniques offer another layer of immediate stress relief. Splashing cold water on your face can provide a shocking yet refreshing jolt that helps reset your system. The cold water stimulates the vagus nerve, which plays a big role in activating the parasympathetic nervous system, promoting relaxation. Using calming scents like lavender or chamomile is also very soothing. Keep an essential oil roller or a small sachet of dried lavender handy, and take a moment to inhale deeply whenever you feel stressed. Listening to soothing music or nature sounds is another powerful sensory technique. Create a playlist of calming tunes or download an app with nature sounds, and take a few minutes to listen and let the stress wash away.

Incorporating these instant stress relief techniques into your daily life can significantly improve your stress management. Whether through breathwork, physical movements, or sensory inputs, these methods provide quick and effective ways to regain control and maintain emotional balance. They are simple, accessible, and can be done anywhere, making them invaluable tools for anyone looking to release trauma, stress, and emotional tension stored in the body.

DAILY STRESS MANAGEMENT ROUTINE

Establishing a daily stress management routine can be a game-changer. When you have a consistent routine, you build resilience to stress by creating a sense of predictability and control in your life. This predictability helps your mind and body know what to expect, reducing the overall impact of stress. Moreover, a structured routine enhances emotional stability, allowing you to easily navigate life's ups and downs. Think about it as setting the stage for a calmer, more balanced day every day.

Start your day with grounding exercises to anchor yourself. These exercises help you feel present and connected to your body. For instance, begin with a simple grounding practice, like feeling your feet on the floor. Stand tall, close your eyes, and shift your weight gently from side to side. Feel the contact between your feet and the ground. This small act can make a big difference, setting a relaxed and positive tone for the day ahead. You might follow this with slow, deliberate stretches, reaching your arms overhead and taking a few deep breaths.

Midday breathwork sessions can be a lifesaver. During lunchtime or a short break, find a quiet spot to sit comfortably and engage in deep breathing exercises to reset and recharge:

1. Inhale deeply through your nose.
2. Hold for a count of three seconds.
3. Exhale slowly through your mouth.
4. Repeat this for a few minutes.

This practice helps to regulate your nervous system, reducing the buildup of stress that can accumulate as the day progresses. It's like hitting the reset button, giving yourself a fresh start even in the middle of a busy day.

Evening relaxation techniques are vital for winding down and preparing for restful sleep. As the day ends, engage in activities that promote relaxation. Gentle yoga stretches can help ease tension in your muscles. Poses like Child's Pose or Legs-Up-the-Wall are particularly soothing. Pair these stretches with deep, calming breaths. Another effective technique is progressive muscle relaxation. Lie down in a comfortable position, and slowly tense and release each muscle from your toes to your head. This practice helps you relax physically and signals to your mind that it's time to unwind.

Incorporating mindfulness practices throughout your day can significantly enhance your stress management routine. Mindful walking is a straightforward but impactful activity. While you walk, pay attention to how your feet connect with the ground, the pattern of your breathing, and the visual and auditory environment surrounding you. This brings you into the present moment, reducing anxiety and promoting calm. Mindful eating is another practice to consider. Take time to taste each bite, noticing the flavors, textures, and aromas of your food. This enhances your eating experience and helps regulate your body's stress response. Body scan meditation is perfect for bedtime. Lie down comfortably, close your eyes, and mentally scan your body from head to toe to become aware of any areas of tension and consciously relax them.

Maintaining consistency in your daily routine can be challenging, but it's crucial for long-term benefits. Setting daily reminders can help keep you on track. Use your phone or a planner to schedule your grounding exercises, breathwork sessions, and relaxation techniques. Keeping a stress management journal is another powerful tool. Note down your practices, how you feel before and after, and any insights you gain. This not only helps you stay accountable but also allows you to track your progress. Adjusting your routine to fit changing schedules is also important. Life is unpredictable, and flexibility is key. If you miss a session, don't stress—simply pick up where you left off and keep going.

Incorporating these practices into your daily life can transform how you handle stress, making you more resilient and emotionally stable.

SOMATIC EXERCISES FOR WORKPLACE STRESS

Workplace stress is a common problem that affects countless individuals across various professions. High workloads and tight deadlines often create a pressure cooker environment, leading to chronic stress and burnout. When you're constantly juggling multiple tasks and racing against the clock, your body and mind bear the brunt. In addition to this, interpersonal conflicts can arise in a collaborative setting, and stress multiplies. The lack of control or autonomy over your work can further exacerbate the situation, making you feel trapped and overwhelmed. This toxic cocktail of stressors impacts your health and hampers your productivity and overall job satisfaction.

To counteract these stressors, incorporating somatic exercises into your workday can be incredibly beneficial.

One effective exercise is the **Seated Spinal Twist**, which you can do right at your desk:

1. Sit up straight with your feet flat on the ground.
2. Place your right hand on the back of your chair.
3. Place your left hand on your right knee.
4. Softly twist your torso to the right, holding the position for a few breaths.
5. Repeat on the other side.

This movement helps release tension in the spine and improves mobility.

Chair yoga poses are another excellent option. Try the **Seated Cat-Cow Stretch**:

1. Sit on the edge of the chair with your hands on your knees.
2. Inhale, arch your back, and look upwards (cow pose).

3. Exhale, round your back, and tuck your chin toward your chest (cat pose).
4. Repeat several times to stretch your back and relieve tension.
5. Wrist and hand stretches are also crucial, especially if you spend a lot of time typing.
6. Extend one arm in front of you with your palm facing up.
7. Use your other hand to softly pull back on your fingers, stretching the wrist and forearm.
8. Hold for a few seconds and switch sides.

These exercises can alleviate the strain from repetitive motions and improve circulation.

In addition to desk-based exercises, taking short movement breaks throughout the day can significantly decrease stress. Standing stretches every hour can help counteract the effects of prolonged sitting. Simply stand up, reach your arms overhead, and stretch your entire body. This quick movement boosts blood flow and energizes your muscles. A quick walk around the office or going outside for a breath of fresh air can also work wonders. Even a five-minute stroll can clear your mind and refresh your energy levels.

If you have a bit more space, consider trying office-friendly Tai Chi movements. These slow, deliberate movements promote relaxation and improve focus.

For example, try the **"Wave Hands Like Clouds"** movement:

1. Stand with your feet shoulder-width apart.
2. slowly shift your weight from one foot to the other while moving your arms in a gentle, waving motion.

This exercise is calming and can be done discreetly in an office setting.

Creating a stress-reducing work environment goes beyond just exercises. An ergonomic desk setup is fundamental. Ensure that your chair supports your lower back and that the computer screen remains at eye level to maintain proper posture. Adding plants and natural elements into your workspace can also have a calming effect. Studies have shown that having greenery around can reduce stress and improve mood. Keeping your workspace tidy and organized is another simple yet effective strategy. A clutter-free environment promotes mental clarity and reduces feelings of overwhelm. Consider using organizers or other storage solutions to keep your desk neat and orderly.

By integrating these somatic exercises and environmental adjustments into your workday, you can create a more balanced and stress-free professional life. These practices improve your physical well-being and enhance your mental clarity and productivity. They are simple and practical and can be seamlessly incorporated into even the busiest of workdays, making them invaluable tools for anyone looking to reduce workplace stress and improve overall well-being.

SELF-COMPASSION PRACTICES TO PREVENT BURNOUT

Self-compassion is a powerful antidote to burnout. At its core, self-compassion involves being kind to yourself, recognizing that you are not alone in your struggles, and practicing mindfulness. It's about treating yourself with the same kindness and understanding you would offer a dear friend. When you're kind to yourself, you create a supportive internal environment that helps you cope with stress and recover from setbacks. Recognizing shared humanity means understanding that everyone makes mistakes and faces challenges. This perspective helps you feel less isolated and more connected to others. Mindfulness, the practice of being present without judgment, allows you to watch and monitor your thoughts and feelings with curiosity rather than criticism. Together, these elements form a robust framework for preventing burnout.

One effective self-compassion exercise is self-compassionate letter writing. Set aside some quiet time, grab a pen and paper, and write to yourself as if you were comforting a friend. Address any mistakes or challenges you're facing with kindness and understanding. Acknowledge your feelings and remember that it's okay to be imperfect. This exercise is incredibly healing, as it shifts your internal dialogue from self-criticism to self-support. Another powerful practice is loving-kindness meditation. Find a comfy position and close your eyes. Begin by focusing on your breath, then softly repeat phrases like, " I will be happy, I will be healthy, I will be safe, I will live with ease." Gradually extend these wishes to others, starting with loved ones and eventually including all beings. This meditation fosters a sense of connection and compassion. Self-compassion breaks are another simple yet effective tool. Throughout your day, take short pauses to offer yourself kindness. Place your hand on your heart, take a few deep breaths, and silently say, "It's okay. I'm doing my best." These moments of self-kindness can help you stay grounded and resilient.

Positive self-talk plays a significant role in enhancing self-compassion and preventing burnout. Reframing negative thoughts is a key technique. When you catch yourself thinking, "I'm not good enough," try to reframe it to, "I'm doing the best I can, and that's enough." This shift in mindset can prevent feelings of inadequacy and boost your self-esteem. Using affirmations is another effective strategy. Create a list of positive statements, such as "I am worthy of love and respect" or "I deserve to take care of myself." Repeat these affirmations daily, especially during challenging moments. Practicing self-encouragement is also crucial. Instead of focusing on what you haven't achieved, celebrate your small wins. Remind yourself of your strengths and the progress you've made. This practice builds resilience and fosters a positive mindset.

Self-compassion routines in your daily life are essential for long-term well-being. Setting aside time for self-care is a fundamental step. Whether reading a book, taking a walk, or enjoying a hobby, prioritize self-care. Creating a self-compassion ritual can also be beneficial. This could be a morning routine that includes meditation, journaling, and setting positive intentions for the day. Having a dedicated time for self-compassion helps reinforce its importance and ensures it becomes a regular practice. Keeping a self-compassion journal is another powerful tool. Each day, write down moments when you were kind to yourself, how you felt, and any insights you gained. This journal is a real reminder of your commitment to self-compassion and allows you to track your progress.

Adding these self-compassion practices into your daily routine can significantly reduce stress and prevent burnout. They create a supportive internal environment that nurtures resilience and well-being. As we wrap up this chapter, remember that self-compassion is not a one-time event but a continuous practice. It's about being kind to yourself, recognizing that you are not alone in your struggles, and staying present without judgment. These practices can transform how you handle stress, making you more resilient and emotionally stable.

CHAPTER 7

SOMATIC EXERCISES

Stress & Burnout

CHAPTER 8
RESTORING GUT HEALTH AND DIGESTION NATURALLY

ABDOMINAL BREATHING FOR DIGESTIVE HEALTH

Abdominal breathing plays a significant role in improving digestion by stimulating the body's natural processes. By practicing deep, diaphragmatic breathing, you stimulate the parasympathetic nervous system, which is also known as the "rest and digest" function. This stimulation promotes peristalsis, the rhythmic movements that propel food through your digestive system. By promoting these movements, abdominal breathing can alleviate issues like bloating and constipation. Additionally, it reduces digestive stress by relaxing the muscles in your intestines, making your digestive system more efficient and comfortable.

Let's start with some basic abdominal breathing techniques that can help better your gut health. **Diaphragmatic breathing (belly breathing)** is a simple yet effective method:

1. Sit or lie down comfortably.
2. Place one hand on your chest and the other on your abdomen.

3. Inhale fully through your nose and let your abdomen rise while your chest remains still.
4. Exhale slowly through your mouth and feel your abdomen fall.

This technique helps manage stress and improves gut health by stimulating the vagus nerve, which regulates digestive functions.

Another beneficial technique is the **4-7-8 Breathing Method**. This exercise can be particularly useful before meals to prepare your digestive system:

1. Sit comfortably and close your eyes.
2. Inhale through your nose for four seconds.
3. Hold your breath for seven seconds.
4. Exhale through your mouth for eight seconds.
5. Repeat this cycle a few more times while focusing on the rhythm of your breath.

This method calms your mind and primes your digestive system for optimal performance.

If you are familiar with basic abdominal breathing, you might want to explore more advanced techniques like the **Three-Part Breath (Dirga Pranayama)**:

1. Divide your inhalation into three parts.
2. First, fill your lower abdomen.
3. Second, fill your mid-abdomen.
4. Third, fill your chest.
5. Exhale in reverse order, emptying your chest, mid-abdomen, and lower abdomen.

This comprehensive approach ensures that your entire respiratory system is engaged, providing a deeper sense of relaxation and aiding digestion.

Breath Retention Techniques (Kumbhaka) can also be beneficial:

1. Start with a deep diaphragmatic breath.
2. Hold your breath for a few seconds, and proceed to exhale slowly.
3. Gradually increase the duration of the breath holds as you become more comfortable.

This technique enhances oxygenation and promotes a calming effect on your digestive system.

Incorporating these breathing exercises into your daily routine can significantly improve your digestive health. Try practicing abdominal breathing before meals to prepare your digestive system. This can help alleviate post-meal discomfort and improve nutrient absorption. Morning and evening abdominal breathing sessions can also set a calming tone for your day and promote relaxation before sleep.

Practical integration of these techniques can be straightforward. Before each meal, take a few minutes to practice diaphragmatic breathing, allowing your body to shift into a relaxed state. If you experience discomfort after eating, try the 4-7-8 breathing method to ease bloating and tension. Starting your day with a few rounds of the Three-Part Breath can invigorate your digestive system, while evening sessions of breath retention techniques can help you create a relaxing night's sleep.

GENTLE MOVEMENTS TO EASE DIGESTIVE DISCOMFORT

Let's talk about the importance of movement for digestion. Gentle physical movements can significantly alleviate digestive discomfort and enhance gut motility. When you engage in specific exercises, you encourage peristalsis, the function that moves food through your digestive tract. This can help reduce gas and bloating, common issues that arise from sluggish digestion. Moreover, regular movement promotes overall digestive health by increasing blood flow to the digestive organs, making sure they function optimally.

One effective movement is the **Seated Spinal Twist**:

1. Sit on the floor or in a chair, keeping your back straight.
2. Place your right hand on your left knee and your left hand behind you for support.
3. Softly twist your torso to the left, looking over your left shoulder.
4. Hold this position for a few breaths, then switch sides.

This twist massages your internal organs and encourages the movement of food and gas through your intestines, helping to relieve bloating and discomfort.

Cat-Cow Stretches are another fantastic option:

1. Begin on your hands and knees.
2. Align your wrists under your shoulders and knees under your hips.
3. Inhale as you arch your back.
4. Lift your head and tailbone up to the ceiling (Cow Pose).
5. Exhale as you round your spine.

6. Tuck your chin to your chest and bring your belly button up to your spine (Cat Pose).
7. Repeat this sequence several times.

This movement stretches the belly muscles and stimulates the intestines, promoting gut motility and easing tension.

Gentle-Forward Bends can also be very soothing for the digestive system:

1. Stand with your feet hip-width apart.
2. Gently bend forward at the hips, letting your upper body hang down.
3. If needed, bend your knees slightly for comfort.
4. Hold onto your elbows and let your head hang heavy.

This pose massages the abdominal organs and can relieve gas and bloating by encouraging the release of trapped air. Incorporating yoga poses specifically designed for digestion can further enhance these benefits.

Wind-Relieving Pose (Pavanamuktasana) is excellent for releasing gas and easing abdominal tension:

1. Lie on your back and bring your knees toward your chest.
2. Hug your knees with your arms, lifting your head and shoulders off the ground if comfortable.
3. Rock gently side to side to massage your lower back and intestines.

Child's Pose (Balasana) is another gentle yoga pose that can aid digestion:

1. Kneel on the floor.
2. Sit back on your heels.

3. Extend your arms forward while lowering your chest to the ground.

This pose relaxes the lower back and abdomen, promoting a sense of calm and easing digestive discomfort.

Bridge Pose (Setu Bandhasana) can also be beneficial:

1. Lie on your back with your knees bent and feet on the floor, hip-width apart.
2. Press into your feet to lift your hips towards the ceiling to create a gentle arch in your back.
3. This pose stimulates the abdominal organs and enhances circulation, supporting overall digestive health.

When practicing these movements, it's crucial to listen to your body and avoid overextension. Modify poses for comfort, using props like pillows or blankets if needed. Practicing these movements after meals can help ease post-meal discomfort and promote better digestion.

SOMATIC PRACTICES FOR GUT-BRAIN CONNECTION

The relationship between your digestive system and your brain is more intricate than you might think. This connection, often called the gut-brain axis, involves constant communication between the two systems. The vagus nerve plays a noteworthy role in this dialogue, acting as a communication highway that sends signals back and forth. When you experience stress or intense emotions, it can directly impact your digestion, leading to issues like stomach aches, bloating, or even irritable bowel syndrome (IBS). Conversely, a troubled digestive system can influence your mood, contributing to anxiety or depression.

CHAPTER 8

To strengthen this gut-brain connection, somatic practices can be highly effective. One such technique is vagal nerve stimulation, which can be achieved through simple activities like humming, singing, or even gargling water. These actions stimulate the vagus nerve, promoting relaxation and enhancing digestive function. Another beneficial practice is a body scan focused on the abdomen. Lie down comfortably and close your eyes. Slowly move your attention from your head to your toes, but spend extra time focusing on your abdomen. Notice any sensations, tension, or discomfort, and breathe into those areas to help release them.

Gut-directed mindfulness meditation is another powerful tool. Sit quietly and place your hands on your abdomen. Close your eyes and take deep, mindful breaths. As you inhale, imagine your breath reaching your digestive organs, bringing with it a sense of calm and healing. As you exhale, visualize any tension or discomfort leaving your body. This practice soothes your digestive system and helps you be more attuned to your body, fostering a deeper connection between your gut and brain.

Visualization techniques can also improve digestive health by creating a positive mental image of your gut. Try visualizing a calm, functioning digestive system. Imagine your stomach and intestines working smoothly like a well-oiled machine. Picture your gut as a place of balance and harmony, where everything flows effortlessly. These positive mental images can have a profound impact on your physical reality, promoting better digestion and overall well-being.

To support the gut-brain connection in daily life, start by eating mindfully and slowly. Make sure to fully chew your food and enjoy every bite. This practice helps with digestion and enables your brain to recognize when you're full, helping you avoid overeating. Practicing gratitude before meals can also set a positive tone. Take a moment to appreciate the food in front of you, acknowledging the effort that went into preparing it. This simple act can enhance your dining experience and promote digestive health.

Adding relaxation techniques into your daily routine can make a significant difference. Whether it's a few minutes of deep breathing, a short meditation session, or even a gentle walk, these activities can help relieve stress and improve gut function. By nurturing the gut-brain connection, you enhance your digestive health and create a more balanced and harmonious state of being.

YOGA POSES FOR GUT HEALTH

Yoga can be an incredible ally for your digestive health, providing both physical and mental benefits. Specific yoga poses stimulate the digestive organs by enhancing blood flow, ensuring they function more efficiently. When you increase blood flow to these organs, you help them absorb nutrients better and work more effectively. But it's not just about the physical benefits. Yoga is also good for relaxation and stress relief, which are crucial for a well-functioning digestive system. Pressure can significantly disrupt your digestive system, causing problems such as bloating and unease. Engaging in yoga can help foster a calmer environment that benefits your gut health.

One excellent pose for aiding digestion is the **Seated Forward Bend (Paschimottanasana)**:

1. Sit with your legs stretched in front of you.
2. Inhale deeply, lengthening your spine.
3. Exhale as you bend at your hips, reaching for your feet.
4. If you can't reach your feet, that's okay—rest your hands on your shins or thighs.

The key is to maintain a long spine and breathe deeply. This pose compresses the abdominal organs, stimulating digestion and relieving bloating.

Another beneficial pose for digestion is the **Supine Twist (Supta Matsyendrasana)**:

1. Lie on your back with your knees bent and feet touching the ground.
2. Stretch your arms out to your sides, forming a T-shape.
3. Softly drop both knees to one side while you keep your shoulders flat on the ground.
4. Turn your head in the opposite direction of your knees for a deeper stretch.
5. Hold for a few breaths, and then switch sides.

This twist massages the intestines, encourages peristalsis, and can relieve gas and constipation.

Combining breath with movement in yoga enhances the digestive benefits of these poses. Inhaling and exhaling during each pose helps you stay present and focused, allowing you to fully engage with the practice. For example, in Seated Forward Bend, inhale to stretch your spine and exhale to deepen the stretch. This breath awareness improves the poses' effectiveness and promotes a sense of calm and relaxation.

A structured yoga sequence focused on gut health can be incredibly beneficial. Start with a warm-up using Cat-Cow Pose to activate your digestive organs. Move into the main sequence with a Seated Forward Bend and Supine Twist to stimulate digestion and relieve tension. Finish with Child's Pose to cool down and relax the entire body. Practicing this sequence regularly can support your digestive health and contribute to a more balanced state of being.

DAILY ROUTINE FOR OPTIMAL DIGESTIVE FUNCTION

A consistent daily routine is key for optimal digestive function and overall gut health. Regularity in meals and practices creates a sense of predictability for your digestive system, allowing it to function more efficiently. When you eat, move, and relax at consistent times each day, your body learns to anticipate these activities, leading to smoother digestion and fewer digestive issues. Think of your digestive system as a well-tuned orchestra that performs best when it follows a regular schedule.

A structured daily routine integrating somatic exercises can support your digestive health. Start your morning with abdominal breathing exercises. Find a quiet spot, sit comfortably, and practice deep, diaphragmatic breathing for five to ten minutes. This sets a calming tone for your day and prepares your digestive system for future meals. Midday is an ideal time for gentle movements. Take a break from your routine and do a few seated spinal twists or a short walk. These activities can stimulate digestion, especially after lunch. In the evening, focus on gut-brain connection practices. Spend a few minutes on a body scan or gut-directed mindfulness meditation to wind down and promote digestive harmony.

In addition to somatic exercises, dietary and lifestyle choices play a crucial role in digestive health. Staying hydrated is paramount. Consuming sufficient water during the day supports a healthy digestive system and helps avoid constipation. Attempt to drink a minimum of eight glasses of water each day. Maintaining a well-rounded diet that is high in fiber is important. Make sure to add a variety of fruits, vegetables, whole grains, and legumes to your food plan. Fiber helps promote consistent bowel movements and contributes to a healthy gut microbiome. On the flip side, avoid common digestive irritants like caffeine, processed foods, and

CHAPTER 8

excessive sugar. These can disrupt your digestive balance and lead to discomfort.

Maintaining consistency in your routine can be challenging, but some strategies can help. Setting reminders for your practices ensures you don't forget to take those vital moments for your health. Use your phone or a planner to schedule times for abdominal breathing, gentle movements, and mindfulness practices. Keeping a digestive health journal can also be beneficial. Note down what you eat, how you feel, and any digestive issues you experience. This can help you identify patterns and make necessary adjustments. Finally, be flexible and adjust your routine to fit your individual needs and schedule. If something isn't working, don't be afraid to tweak it until you find what suits you best.

Incorporating these practices into your daily life can transform your digestive health. You can support a healthy, well-functioning digestive system by creating a consistent routine, making mindful dietary choices, and staying committed. This balance not only benefits your gut but also enhances your overall well-being.

CHAPTER 8

SOMATIC EXERCISES

BONUS: Weight Loss Help

CHAPTER 9
BETTER SLEEP THROUGH DEEP RELAXATION AND BREATHWORK

WIND-DOWN ROUTINE FOR BETTER SLEEP

A well-structured wind-down routine can be a game-changer for your sleep quality. By engaging in calming activities before sleeping, you signal to your body that it's time to wind down. This routine plays a crucial role in setting your circadian rhythms, the internal clock that regulates your sleep-wake cycle. When you consistently follow a pre-sleep routine, your body learns to recognize these cues, making it easier to sleep and wake up at regular times. This consistency helps you sleep better and reduces pre-sleep anxiety, creating a smoother transition from wakefulness to slumber.

Gentle Evening Stretches are a wonderful addition to any wind-down routine. These stretches help relax your muscles and release the day's tension, preparing your body for rest:

- Start with forward bends.
- Stand with your feet hip-width apart and bend at the hips.
- Let your upper body hang down.

This stretch releases tension in your back and shoulders, promoting relaxation. Next, move into **Child's Pose (Balasana)**:

1. Kneel on the floor.
2. Sit back on your heels.
3. Extend your arms forward.
4. Lower your chest to the ground.

This gentle pose stretches your lower back and hips, creating a sense of calm. Finally, try the **Legs-Up-the-Wall Pose (Viparita Karani)**:

1. Lie on your back.
2. Extend your legs up against a wall.

This pose encourages blood flow away from your legs and calms the nervous system, making it easier to drift off to sleep.

Incorporating relaxation techniques into your wind-down routine can further enhance its effectiveness. Progressive muscle relaxation is a practice where you tighten and then gradually let go of various muscle groups. Begin at your toes and move upward to your head, contracting each muscle group for a few seconds before relaxing. This approach aids in alleviating physical tension and encourages a state of relaxation. Gentle yoga nidra, a form of guided meditation, can also be incredibly soothing. Lie down in a comfortable position and follow a guided session that takes you through various stages of relaxation, helping to calm the mind and body.

Another excellent technique is a guided **Body Scan Meditation**:

1. Lie down.
2. Close your eyes.
3. Mentally scan your body from head to toe.
4. Relax any tension-filled area you notice.

Creating an effective wind-down routine involves several practical steps. Begin by establishing a regular bedtime. Sleeping at the same hour each night helps stabilize your internal clock. Limit screen time for at least an hour before sleeping, as the blue light from devices such as phones, tablets, and computers can disrupt your body's melatonin production, which is essential for sleep. Instead, participate in soothing activities like reading a physical book or listening to soft music. Calming scents, such as chamomile, can also further enhance your wind-down routine. You might consider using essential oils in a diffuser or lighting a scented candle to foster a relaxing environment.

Treating your wind-down routine as a non-negotiable part of your day can help ensure you stick to it. Just like brushing your teeth or having dinner, make your wind-down activities a regular habit. Over time, your body will come to recognize these cues, making it easier to transition from the busyness of the day to the tranquility of sleep.

BEDTIME BREATHWORK PRACTICES

Breathwork can play a powerful role in preparing your body for sleep. By engaging in specific breathing exercises, you can activate the parasympathetic nervous system, the section of your nervous system in charge of rest and digestion. This activation helps reduce your heart rate and blood pressure, creating a calming effect that makes it easier to fall asleep. As your mind quiets down, anxiety and stress begin to fade, making room for peaceful slumber. Breathwork is not just about breathing deeply; it's about directing your breath in a way that signals your body to relax fully.

One of the simplest and most effective techniques is **Extended Exhalation Breathing**, which focuses on lengthening the exhale to promote relaxation:

1. Sit or lie down in a comfortable position and close your eyes.
2. Begin by taking a full breath in through your nose for four seconds.
3. Exhale calmly through your mouth for a count of eight.

The extended exhale helps activate the parasympathetic nervous system, promoting a sense of calm. Focus on the feeling of the breath leaving your body as you repeat this cycle.

Equal breathing (Sama Vritti) is another simple yet powerful breathwork practice. This technique involves making your inhales and exhales the same length:

1. Sit or lie down comfortably and close your eyes.
2. Inhale through your nose for four seconds.
3. Exhale through your nose for four seconds.

This balanced breathing pattern helps to steady the mind and body, creating a sense of equilibrium that is conducive to sleep. You can start with a count of four and gradually increase to a count of six or eight as you become more comfortable with the practice.

Integrating breathwork into your bedtime routine can be seamless and straightforward. You can practice these techniques while lying in bed, making it easy to transition from daytime activities to sleep. Combining breathwork with visualization can enhance its calming effects. For instance, while practicing extended exhalation breathing, you can visualize a serene beach or a peaceful forest. Using breathwork as a bridge from your daily activities to your wind-down routine can help signal to your body that it's time to relax and wind down to sleep.

CHAPTER 9

SOMATIC EXERCISES TO COMBAT INSOMNIA

Insomnia can feel like a relentless foe, robbing you of the rest you desperately need. The good news is that somatic exercises can be a powerful ally in your fight against sleepless nights. These exercises work by regulating the nervous system, which plays a crucial role in prepping your body for sleep. You can activate the parasympathetic nervous system by engaging in specific movements, promoting relaxation. This activation helps reduce the adrenaline and cortisol levels that keep you alert, making it easier to drift off.

Physical tension often accumulates in our bodies throughout the day, contributing to insomnia. Somatic exercises can help release this tension, making your body feel more relaxed and ready for sleep. For instance, **Gentle Spine Twists** can be incredibly effective:

1. Lie on your back with your arms stretched out to the sides.
2. Bend your knees and drop them to one side while turning your head to the opposite side.
3. Hold this position for a few breaths, then switch sides.

This simple movement helps release tension in the spine and lower back, creating a sense of ease.

Pelvic Tilts are another excellent exercise for combating insomnia:

1. Lie on your back with your knees bent and feet on the ground.
2. Slowly tilt your pelvis upward, pressing your lower back into the ground, then release.
3. Repeat this movement several times, focusing on the gentle rocking motion.

Pelvic tilts help release tension in the lower back and hips, areas where stress often accumulates. This exercise can make your body feel more comfortable and ready for sleep.

The **Butterfly Stretch** is also beneficial for promoting relaxation:

1. Sit on the floor with your feet together and your knees bent out to the sides.
2. Hold your feet with your hands and softly press your knees down towards the floor.
3. You will feel a stretch in your inner thighs and hips.
4. Hold this position for a few breaths, then release.

The butterfly stretch helps open up the hips and release tension, creating a feeling of openness and ease.

Combining mindfulness practices with somatic exercises can enhance their effectiveness. Mindful movement sequences encourage you to stay present and aware of your body's sensations. For example, as you perform gentle spine twists or pelvic tilts, focus on the feeling of your muscles stretching and relaxing. Notice your breath, inhaling deeply and exhaling calmly. This mindful awareness helps deepen the relaxation response, making it easier for your body to transition into sleep.

Breath awareness can also be integrated into your somatic exercises. As you perform movements like the butterfly stretch, focus on synchronizing your breath with your actions. Inhale deeply as you prepare to stretch, and exhale slowly as you ease into the position. The integration of breathing and movement aids in soothing the nervous system and alleviating anxiety, which facilitates falling asleep more easily.

A body scan during somatic exercises can be a powerful tool for combating insomnia. As you move through different stretches and movements, take a moment to mentally scan your body from head to toe. Take note of any areas of tension or discomfort and consciously relax them. This practice helps create a deeper connection between your mind and body, enhancing the relaxation response and preparing you for sleep.

Timing your somatic exercises for maximum benefit is crucial. Aim to practice these exercises 30 minutes to an hour before bed. This timing allows your body to transition from the day's activities to a state of relaxation. Keep the movements gentle and slow, avoiding any exercises that might be too stimulating. Modify the exercises to fit your comfort level, using props like pillows or blankets to support your body as needed.

By adding these practices into your nightly routine, you can create a soothing pre-sleep ritual that helps combat insomnia and promotes restful sleep.

CREATING A SLEEP-FRIENDLY ENVIRONMENT

A peaceful, inviting sleep environment can make a big difference when it comes to getting a good night's sleep. The physical surroundings in your bedroom play a crucial role in how well you sleep. Factors like light, sound, and temperature can significantly impact sleep quality. Bright lights, especially blue light from screens, can slow down melatonin production, making it harder to fall asleep. Meanwhile, a noisy environment can keep you awake or disrupt your sleep cycles. Even the temperature of your room can affect how well you sleep; too hot or too cold, and you'll find yourself waking up throughout the night. Creating the right environment can help signal to your body that it's time to rest, making falling and staying asleep easier.

Think about utilizing blackout curtains or sleep masks to eliminate light and enhance your sleeping atmosphere. Light exposure can disrupt your body's natural sleep cycle, making it much harder to fall asleep and maintain sleep. Blackout curtains are specifically created to prevent outside light from entering, establishing a dark and cozy environment that promotes better sleep. If blackout curtains aren't an option, an eye mask can be a simple yet effective alternative. Keeping your bedroom cool and well-ventilated is also crucial. A temperature between 60-67°F (15-19°C) is generally recommended for optimal sleep. Utilize fans, air conditioning, and open windows to keep a pleasant temperature and promote proper air circulation.

Noise can be another significant barrier to restful sleep. If you live in a noisy area or have a loud household, consider using earplugs or a white noise machine. Earplugs can block out disruptive sounds, while white noise machines generate a consistent, soothing background noise that can mask other sounds. This can help create a calm environment, allowing you to drift off more easily. Some people also find comfort in the sound of nature, such as ocean waves or rain, which can be played through an app or device.

Creating a calming bedtime atmosphere can further enhance your sleep environment. Using calming colors and decor can also promote relaxation. Soft colors and neutrals can promote a serene and inviting space. Incorporating soothing scents such as chamomile can also help signal your body that it's time to wind down. Keeping your bedroom tidy and clutter-free can also make a significant difference. A clean, organized space can promote a sense of calm and relaxation, making it easier to fall asleep.

Maintaining a sleep-friendly environment requires some ongoing effort. Regularly changing and washing your bedding can help create a fresh and inviting space. Clean sheets and pillowcases can enhance your comfort and make your bed more inviting. Keeping phones and other electronics out of the bedroom is also essential. Devices like smartphones, tablets, and TVs emit blue light, which can interfere with your sleep. Consider creating a tech-free bedroom to promote better sleep hygiene. Establishing a consistent

CHAPTER 9

bedtime ritual can also help maintain a sleep-friendly environment. This could include activities such as reading a book, listening to calming music, or gentle relaxation exercises.

Making these changes and maintaining a sleep-conducive environment can significantly improve your sleep quality, helping you wake up feeling refreshed and ready to face the day.

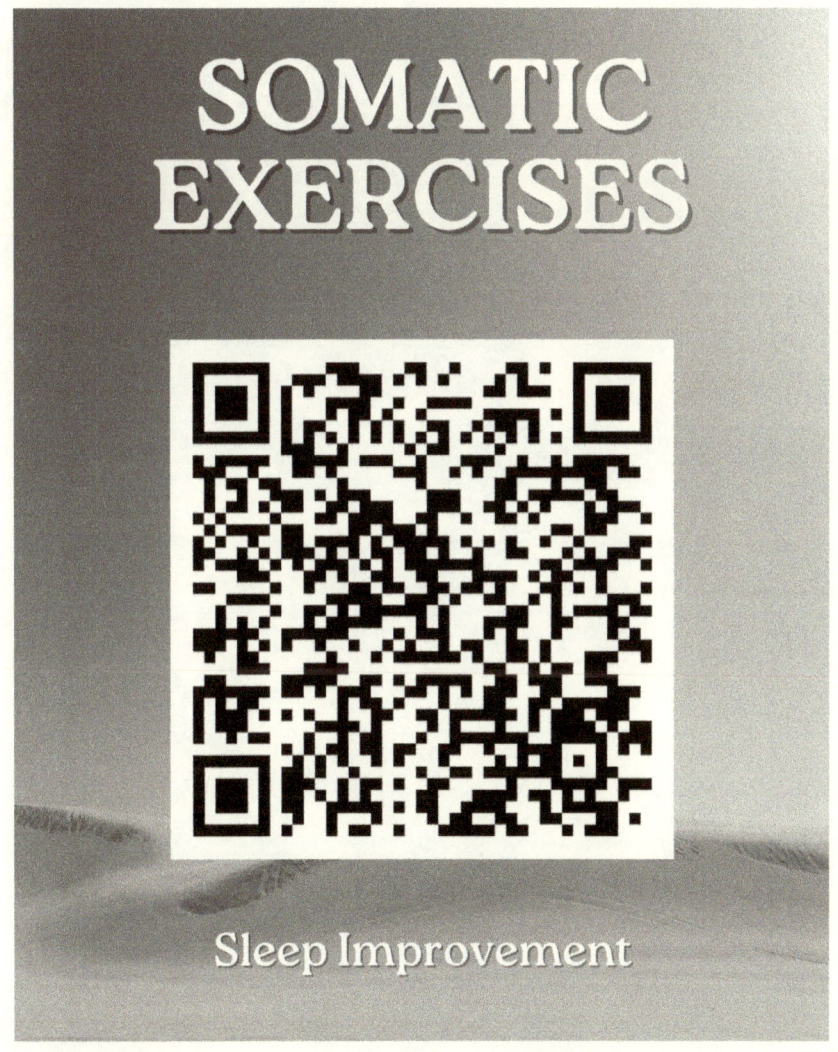

CHAPTER 10
SUPPORT IMMUNITY AND REDUCE INFLAMMATION THROUGH BODY AWARENESS

BREATHWORK FOR IMMUNE SUPPORT

Breathwork can significantly enhance immune function and support overall health. When you engage in specific breathwork practices, you activate the parasympathetic nervous system, which is in charge of promoting relaxation and reducing stress. This activation helps lower stress hormones like cortisol, which, when elevated, can hurt the immune system. Additionally, breathwork improves the oxygenation of tissues, ensuring that your cells receive the oxygen they require to work effectively. This is particularly important for immune cells, which require sufficient oxygen to combat pathogens effectively.

Let's start with some basic immune-supportive breathwork techniques. One of the simplest yet most effective methods is **Deep Diaphragmatic Breathing**:

1. Sit or lie down comfortably.
2. Place one hand on your chest and the other on your stomach.

3. As you inhale deeply through your nose.
4. Allow your stomach to rise while keeping your chest as still as possible.
5. Exhale calmly through your mouth and feel your stomach fall.

This kind of breathing promotes complete oxygen exchange, reduces the heart rate, and can help decrease or stabilize blood pressure.

For those who are comfortable with basic breathwork and looking to explore more advanced techniques, the Wim Hof Method offers a powerful option. This method involves taking 30-40 deep breaths in quick succession, followed by a breath hold and then a deep exhalation. This practice can significantly increase oxygen levels in your body, boost your immune response, and enhance overall resilience.

Another advanced technique is **Skull-Shining Breath (Kapalabhati)**. To perform this exercise:

- Sit comfortably with a straight spine.
- Take a full breath and exhale forcefully through your nose while tightening your abdominal muscles.
- Repeat this for 30-50 breaths.

This technique cleanses the respiratory system and invigorates your mind and body, providing a natural energy boost.

Integrating these breathwork practices into your daily life can be simple and highly effective. Start your day with a morning immune-boosting breathwork session. Spend five to ten minutes practicing deep diaphragmatic breathing or the 4-7-8 technique. This will help set a calm tone for the day ahead. During midday, take short breathwork breaks. A few rounds of Wim Hof breathing or Kapalabhati can revitalize your energy levels and keep your immune system functioning optimally. In the evening, wind down with relaxation breathwork, such as the 4-7-8 technique, to prepare your body for a restful night's sleep.

Daily Breathwork Log

To help you stay consistent, consider keeping a Daily Breathwork Log. Each day, note the technique practiced, the duration, and how you felt before and after the session. Over time, this log will help you identify which techniques work best for you and how they impact your overall well-being.

Here's a printable log book to get you started:

By incorporating these breathwork practices and tracking your progress, you can effectively support your immune system, reduce stress, and improve your overall health.

DAILY ROUTINE FOR IMMUNE HEALTH

Sticking to a consistent daily routine is a game-changer for your immune health and overall well-being. Regularity in immune-supportive practices can create a sense of predictability for your body, making it easier to maintain a balanced and healthy system. When your body knows what to expect, it can function more efficiently, reducing the stress that unpredictability can bring. This predictability can be beneficial for those dealing with chronic stress or trauma stored in the body, as it provides a stable framework within which healing can occur.

To start your day on the right foot, incorporate morning breathwork designed to support immune health. Begin your day with deep diaphragmatic breathing for about five to ten minutes. This practice can set a calm and focused tone, preparing your body to face the day with resilience. Following your breathwork session, engage in a nutritious breakfast rich in antioxidants. Foods like berries, nuts, and green tea can provide a powerful start, fueling your body with essential nutrients that support immune function.

Midday is an excellent time to incorporate gentle movements into your routine. These movements can help alleviate any tension that has built up during the morning and keep your lymphatic system active. Simple stretches, a short walk, or even a quick yoga session can make a difference. If you're at work or have a busy day, take a few minutes to stand up, stretch, and move around. This can improve circulation and decrease the risk of inflammation, which is crucial for maintaining a healthy immune system.

As the day winds down, focus on evening relaxation techniques to prepare your body for a restful night. Practices such as progressive muscle relaxation, gentle yoga stretches, or guided meditation can help signal to your body that it's time to relax and recover. This is also a good time to reflect on your day and note any areas of tension or stress that you might want to address in your future practices. Incorporate a light, nutritious dinner that includes foods with plenty of vitamins and minerals to support your immune system overnight.

In addition to these somatic practices, there are several dietary and lifestyle tips that can complement your routine. Staying hydrated is of utmost importance. Water helps provide nutrients to cells and aids in detoxifying the body. Aim for at least eight glasses of water a day. Maintaining a well-rounded diet that is high in antioxidants is important as well. Add fruits, vegetables, whole grains, and lean proteins into your meals. Avoid common immune suppressors such as sugar and alcohol, as they can weaken your immune response and make you more susceptible to illnesses.

Maintaining consistency in your routine can sometimes be challenging, but there are strategies that can help. Setting reminders for your practices can ensure you stay on track. Use your phone or a planner to schedule your breathwork, movements, and relaxation techniques. Keeping an immune health journal can also be beneficial. Note down what practices you did, how you felt before and after, and any changes you notice in your overall well-being. This can help you identify what works best for you and keep you motivated. Adjust your routine to fit your individual needs and schedules. If you miss a session, don't be hard on yourself; simply pick up where you left off and continue your practice.

Adding these practices into your daily life allows you to create a robust framework that supports your immune health, reduces stress, and enhances your overall well-being.

SOMATIC PRACTICES FOR CHRONIC INFLAMMATION

Chronic inflammation can be a silent but potent adversary, contributing to a range of health conditions such as arthritis, cardiovascular disease, and even some forms of cancer. It's a state where the body's immune response goes into overdrive, producing chemicals that can damage tissues over time. This persistent inflammation can lead to joint pain, fatigue, and other symptoms that can negatively impact your quality of life. Reducing inflammation is crucial for overall well-being, which is where somatic practices come into play. You can effectively manage and reduce chronic inflammation by incorporating specific exercises and mindfulness techniques.

One of the most accessible ways to combat chronic inflammation is through gentle stretching routines. Stretching helps to maintain flexibility, improve circulation, and reduce muscle tension, all of which are beneficial for lowering inflammation.

Start with basic stretches like the **Hamstring Stretch**:

1. Sit on the floor.
2. Extended one leg and the other bent, reaching towards your foot with a straight back.
3. Hold for a few seconds and switch sides.

Another effective stretch is the **Seated Spinal Twist**:

1. Sit with your back straight.
2. Extend one leg and cross the other over it, placing your opposite elbow on the outside of your crossed knee.
3. Twist gently to look over your shoulder.

These stretches are simple yet powerful in maintaining mobility and reducing stiffness.

Restorative yoga poses can also be incredibly effective in managing chronic inflammation. These poses are designed to promote relaxation and stress relief, both of which are needed for reducing inflammatory markers in the body.

Try the **Reclining Bound Angle Pose (Supta Baddha Konasana)**:

1. Lie on your back with the bottom of your feet together and your knees falling open to the sides.
2. Use pillows or props to support your knees if needed.

Another great pose is the **Supported Bridge Pose (Setu Bandhasana)**:

1. Lie on your back with your knees bent.
2. Keep your feet flat on the ground.
3. Lift your hips towards the ceiling.
4. Place a block or cushion under your lower back for support.
5. Hold these poses for several minutes to allow your body to relax and release tension.

Incorporating mindfulness into somatic practices can enhance their effectiveness. Mindful movement sequences, where you focus on each movement's sensations, can deepen your practice. For instance, while performing a simple stretch, pay attention to how your muscles feel, how your skin stretches, and your breath's rhythm. Combining breath awareness with physical stretches can also be beneficial. Inhale deeply as you prepare to stretch, and exhale as you extend into the stretch. This synergy of breath and movement helps to calm the mind and reduce stress. A body scan during somatic exercises can further enhance the practice. As you move through different poses or stretches, mentally scan your body from head to toe, taking note of areas with tension and consciously relaxing them.

Managing chronic inflammation also involves making lifestyle changes. An anti-inflammatory diet can serve as an effective strategy. Prioritize eating foods high in antioxidants, such as berries, leafy greens, and nuts. Omega-3 fatty acids in fish and flaxseeds can likewise aid in minimizing inflammation. Consistent physical activity is essential. Target at least 30 minutes of exercise on most days of the week. Activities like walking, swimming, or gentle yoga can keep inflammation at bay. Methods for managing stress, like meditation, journaling, or enjoying nature, can significantly influence your inflammation levels. Persistent stress is a recognized factor that contributes to inflammation, making it vital to discover effective ways to handle it.

GENTLE MOVEMENTS TO REDUCE INFLAMMATION

Imagine feeling the heavy burden of inflammation in your body, making every movement feel like wading through thick mud. This was the case for Karen, a retired schoolteacher who struggled with chronic pain, especially in her joints. She discovered that gentle physical movements could be a game-changer. These exercises alleviated her symptoms and improved her overall well-being. The importance of movement in reducing inflammation cannot be overstated. Gentle exercises promote lymphatic drainage, which is crucial for flushing out toxins and reducing swelling. They also help lower inflammatory markers in the blood, aiding in the fight against chronic diseases. Moreover, improved circulation and mobility can make everyday tasks feel less daunting and more manageable.

One effective way to promote lymphatic drainage is through specific exercises designed to stimulate the lymphatic system. Start with simple movements like bouncing on the balls of your feet or gently shaking your arms and legs. These actions encourage lymph fluid to move through your body, aiding in detoxification. Gentle joint rotations are also incredibly beneficial. Begin by rotating your wrists, ankles, and neck in slow, controlled circles. This helps reduce stiffness and enhances the flow of synovial fluid, which lubricates your joints. Soft tissue stretches are another excellent way to reduce inflammation. Focus on areas that tend to hold tension, such as your shoulders, back, and hamstrings. Stretching these muscles can alleviate tightness and improve overall flexibility.

Incorporating specific yoga poses can further enhance the benefits of gentle movements in reducing inflammation. Legs-Up-the-Wall Pose, or Viparita Karani, is particularly effective. To do this, lie on your back with your legs extended up against a wall. This pose encourages blood flow away from your legs and reduces swelling.

When practicing these movements, it's crucial to listen to your body and avoid overextension. Stop immediately and modify the exercise to suit your needs if you feel any pain or discomfort. Use props like cushions, blocks, or straps to make poses more accessible and comfortable. Practicing movements slowly and mindfully is key. Focus on your breath and the sensations in your body. This mindful approach not only ensures safe practice but also enhances the calming effects of the exercises.

Inflammation Reduction Checklist

Consider using an Inflammation Reduction Checklist. This simple tool will keep you accountable and ensure you incorporate these gentle movements into your daily routine.

Here's a printable checklist to get you started:

Making these gentle movements a regular part of your routine can significantly reduce inflammation, improve mobility, and enhance your overall quality of life.

CHAPTER 10

SOMATIC EXERCISES

Immune System Support & Inflammation

CHAPTER 11
INTEGRATING SOMATIC PRACTICES INTO DAILY LIFE

TRACKING PROGRESS AND STAYING MOTIVATED

Tracking your progress in somatic practice is like keeping a journal of your journey. It's a way to see how far you've come and to stay motivated. Knowing where you started and noting the changes along the way can be incredibly empowering. When you track your progress, you give yourself a tangible way to measure improvement, which can be particularly motivating when you feel stuck or discouraged. Consistently seeing positive changes can reinforce your commitment to the practice and keep you moving forward.

There are several methods you can use to track your progress. Journaling is one of the most effective tools. By writing down your somatic experiences, you can capture the nuances of your practice, noting how your body feels before and after exercises, any emotional shifts, and any insights you gain. This practice helps you track progress and deepen your self-awareness. Additionally, you can use progress charts and graphs to visualize your improvements. For example, you might track the frequency and duration of your practices or chart changes in specific symptoms like reduced anxiety or improved sleep. Keeping a practice log with dates, types of exercises, and personal reflections can also be beneficial.

Self-reflection plays a key role in understanding your progress and identifying areas for improvement. Regular self-reflection helps you to check in with yourself, providing a moment to pause and consider how you're feeling physically and emotionally. Reflective questions can guide this process: What changes have I noticed in my body? How do I feel after practicing somatic exercises? What challenges have I encountered, and how did I address them? Monthly review sessions can be particularly helpful. Set aside time at the end of each month to review your journal entries, practice logs, and progress charts. Reflect on your achievements, identify patterns, and consider any adjustments you might need to make to your routine. This process can provide valuable insights and help you stay on track.

Staying motivated in your somatic practice requires both short-term and long-term goals. Setting clear, achievable goals can give you something to strive for and a sense of direction. Short-term goals might include practicing a specific exercise daily for a week or focusing on breathwork before bed each night. Long-term goals could involve more substantial changes, like reducing chronic pain or managing anxiety more effectively over several months. Celebrate your milestones and achievements, no matter how small they might seem. Each step forward is progress and deserves to be recognized as a win. Celebrating can be as simple as acknowledging your efforts with a moment of gratitude or treating yourself to something enjoyable.

Seeking support from a somatic community or group can also help maintain your motivation. Surrounding yourself with other people who share similar goals can give you encouragement, accountability, and a sense of connection. This support can be found in local somatic therapy groups, online forums, or social media communities. Sharing your experiences and hearing about others' experiences can inspire you and remind you that you're not alone in this process.

Reflective Journaling Prompts

Consider using these prompts to guide your self-reflection:

- What physical sensations did I notice during my practice today?
- How did my emotional state change before and after the exercises?
- What challenges did I encounter, and how did I address them?
- What progress have I made in the past month?
- What are my goals for the next week/month?

By incorporating progress tracking, self-reflection, and community support into your somatic practice, you can stay motivated and clearly see the benefits of your efforts. This approach enhances your commitment and deepens your connection to the practice, making it a more integral part of your life.

Reflective Journaling Prompts

Prompt: After practicing a somatic exercise, take a few minutes to reflect on your experience. Write about what you felt in your body, any emotions that surfaced, and how the practice impacted your overall state of mind. This exercise can deepen your self-awareness and help you track your progress over time.

ADAPTING EXERCISES TO FIT YOUR LIFESTYLE

Personalizing your somatic exercises to fit your lifestyle is crucial for effectiveness. Everyone's life is different, and a one-size-fits-all approach simply doesn't work. By tailoring your practices to your specific needs, preferences, and limitations, you increase the likelihood of sticking with them and reaping the benefits. Whether you have a busy schedule or physical limitations or prefer certain types of movements, personalization ensures that your somatic exercises are both practical and enjoyable.

Customizing exercises for time constraints can make a significant difference. If you find it hard to carve out long periods for practice, break it down into shorter, more manageable sessions. For example, a busy professional might not have an hour to spare but can fit in quick desk stretches throughout the day. These stretches could include seated spinal twists, shoulder rolls, and neck stretches. Each of these can be done in just a few minutes and can help alleviate tension without disrupting your workday.

Physical limitations are another factor to consider. If you have mobility issues or chronic pain, modify your movements to suit your comfort level. Instead of standing exercises, opt for seated or lying-down versions. For instance, seated cat-cow stretches or lying-down pelvic tilts can provide similar benefits without putting strain on your body. Props like pillows, straps, or blocks can also help make exercises more accessible and comfortable.

Incorporating somatic practices into daily activities can make them feel less like a chore and more like a natural part of your routine. If you're a stay-at-home parent, you can integrate exercises with childcare. While playing with your child on the floor, practice gentle stretches like child's pose or butterfly stretches. These movements can be done while engaging with your child, making it a bonding activity as well.

CHAPTER 11

Retirees might find it easier to create a relaxed practice schedule. Without the pressures of a hectic work life, you can dedicate specific times of the day to somatic exercises. Morning stretches can help wake up the body, while evening relaxation techniques can prepare you for a restful night's sleep. You can also explore different types of somatic practices at a leisurely pace, finding what works best for you.

Staying flexible and adaptable in your practice is key to long-term success. Your body's needs can change daily, so it's important to listen to its signals and make adjustments as needed. If you're feeling particularly tired or sore one day, opt for gentler exercises or shorter sessions. On days when you have more energy, you might choose to engage in more dynamic movements or longer practice sessions. This adaptability ensures your practice remains sustainable and responsive to your body's needs.

Experimenting with new techniques can also keep your practice fresh and engaging. Don't be afraid to try different types of movements or combine them in unique ways. You might discover that a certain combination of stretches and breathwork provides the most relief for your specific tension points. Staying open to new approaches can lead to unexpected benefits and a deeper connection to your practice.

Maintaining flexibility in your routine means being kind to yourself. Life can be unpredictable, and there will be days when your planned practice doesn't happen. Rather than feeling discouraged, recognize that it's okay to miss a session and return to your routine when possible. Consistency is important, but so is understanding that self-care is about progress, not perfection.

CASE STUDIES: REAL-LIFE APPLICATIONS AND SUCCESSES

Case studies are invaluable for understanding somatic exercises' real-world application and success. They provide detailed insights into how these practices work in various contexts, offering concrete evidence of their effectiveness. By examining individual experiences, you can understand how somatic therapy can be tailored to address specific needs and challenges. This section will delve into several well-documented case studies, highlighting the practical techniques and measurable outcomes.

Consider the case of Jack, a military veteran who struggled with PTSD after returning from service. Traditional therapies had provided some relief, but he continued to experience flashbacks, hypervigilance, and emotional numbness. Jack's therapist introduced him to trauma release exercises (TRE), a somatic practice designed to help the body release deep muscular stress and trauma. Through a series of guided exercises, such as leg lifts and gentle shaking, Jack was able to access and release the stored tension in his body. Over time, he noticed a significant reduction in his PTSD symptoms. He experienced fewer flashbacks, felt more present in his daily life, and began to reconnect with his emotions. Jack's journey illustrates how somatic therapy can offer profound relief for trauma survivors by addressing the physical manifestations of their experiences.

In another case, we have Emily, a corporate employee who faced constant workplace stress. The high demands of her job left her feeling overwhelmed and physically tense. Emily incorporated somatic routines into her daily schedule, starting with desk-friendly stretches and breathwork. She practiced simple exercises like shoulder rolls and neck stretches, combined with 4-7-8 breathing, multiple times throughout the day. These quick, accessible techniques helped Emily manage her stress levels more effectively.

CHAPTER 11

She reported enhanced productivity, reduced stress, and a greater sense of well-being. By integrating somatic exercises into her workday, Emily was able to create a more balanced and productive professional life.

Then there's Alex, a teenager who struggles with emotional regulation. He often felt overwhelmed by his emotions, leading to frequent outbursts and a sense of instability. Alex's therapist introduced him to grounding techniques, body scans, and somatic practices designed to help people reconnect with their bodies and regulate their emotions. Alex started with simple grounding exercises, like feeling his feet on the ground and focusing on the sensations in his body. He also practiced body scans, where he would mentally scan his body from head to toe, noting areas of tension and consciously relaxing them. These practices helped Alex develop greater emotional stability and resilience.

The specific techniques used in these case studies varied, but all shared a common goal: to help individuals release stored tension and reconnect with their bodies. In Jack's case, trauma release exercises (TRE) were instrumental in his recovery. These exercises focus on evoking natural tremors in the body, which help release deep-seated stress and trauma. For Emily, desk-friendly stretches like shoulder rolls, neck stretches, and breathwork provided quick and effective stress relief throughout her workday. Alex benefited from grounding techniques and body scans, which helped him develop a greater awareness of his body and emotions.

The measurable outcomes and benefits experienced by these individuals are significant. Jack saw a reduction in trauma-related symptoms, such as flashbacks and hypervigilance, which improved his overall quality of life. Emily found that her enhanced productivity and reduced stress levels made her workday more manageable and enjoyable. Alex's improved emotional stability and resilience allowed him to navigate the challenges of adolescence easier.

These case studies highlight the potential of somatic exercises. They show that these practices can be tailored made to meet the specific needs of individuals, providing you with an effective approach to healing. Whether you are dealing with trauma, workplace stress, or emotional regulation issues, somatic exercises provide practical tools to help you release stored tension and improve your overall well-being.

By adapting somatic exercises to fit your lifestyle, you create a practice that is both effective and sustainable. Whether you're a busy professional fitting in quick stretches, a stay-at-home parent integrating exercises with childcare, or a retiree exploring new techniques at a relaxed pace, personalization ensures that your practice meets your unique needs. This approach not only enhances the effectiveness of the exercises but also makes them a more enjoyable and integral part of your daily life.

CONCLUSION

You've embarked on a journey through the world of somatic therapy, exploring its profound impact on healing trauma, relieving stress, and regulating your nervous system. The essence of somatic treatment lies in its ability to reconnect the mind and body, offering a holistic approach to well-being. By focusing on bodily sensations and movements, somatic exercises help release stored tension and promote emotional and physical health.

Throughout this book, we've delved into various somatic exercises, including breathwork, body scans, gentle movements, grounding techniques, and visualization practices. Each of these exercises offers unique benefits, catering to different needs and conditions. Breathwork enhances your body's natural relaxation response, body scans increase awareness of physical sensations, and gentle movements alleviate physical tension. Grounding techniques anchor you in the present moment, while visualization practices foster a sense of calm and safety.

The benefits of somatic exercises are vast and varied. For chronic pain patients, these practices can provide much-needed relief by reducing muscle tension and improving flexibility. Emotional regu-

CONCLUSION

lation becomes more manageable as you learn to recognize and process your feelings through somatic awareness. Sleep quality improves with routines that prepare your body and mind for rest. Trauma survivors find solace in exercises that help them reconnect with their bodies and let go of pent-up emotions. Integrating somatic practices into your daily life is crucial for sustained benefits. Consistency is key. Regular practice ensures that the positive effects of somatic exercises become ingrained in your routine, leading to long-term improvements in mental, emotional, and physical health. Think of it as a daily commitment to yourself, a gift of self-care that pays off in profound ways.

Somatic therapy's holistic approach addresses mental, emotional, and physical well-being. It's not just about alleviating symptoms but nurturing overall resilience and strength. By engaging in these practices, you equip yourself with tools to navigate life's challenges with greater ease and grace. Remember, personalization is essential. Tailor your somatic practice to fit your unique lifestyle and needs. Whether you're a busy professional, a stay-at-home parent, or someone with physical limitations, there's a way to make these exercises work for you. Flexibility and adaptability ensure that your practice remains enjoyable and effective.

Self-compassion and mindfulness are vital components of your healing journey. Be kind to yourself, acknowledge your progress, and understand that healing is not linear. There will be ups and downs, but every small step forward is significant. Set personal goals and intentions to keep yourself motivated and focused. Consider joining a community or finding a support group to share experiences and receive encouragement. There's strength in numbers, and knowing you're not alone can be incredibly empowering. Revisit this book and refer back to specific chapters as needed. Healing is an ongoing journey, and it's okay to seek guidance and reinforcement along the way.

CONCLUSION

Thank you for choosing this book and trusting me to guide your healing journey. Your commitment and courage in taking steps toward better mental, emotional, and physical health are commendable. Continue exploring and learning about new techniques and approaches to enhance your somatic practice. The world of somatic therapy is vast, and there's always more to discover. Remember, healing is an ongoing journey. Every small step you take is significant. Embrace the process and celebrate your progress, no matter how small it may seem. Your resilience and dedication have the power to transform your life.

As you move forward, hold onto the belief that you have the strength and capacity to heal. Somatic therapy offers a path to greater self-awareness, emotional balance, and physical well-being. Embrace this journey with an open heart and mind, and know that you are capable of profound transformation.

Wishing you peace, resilience, and continued growth on your healing journey.

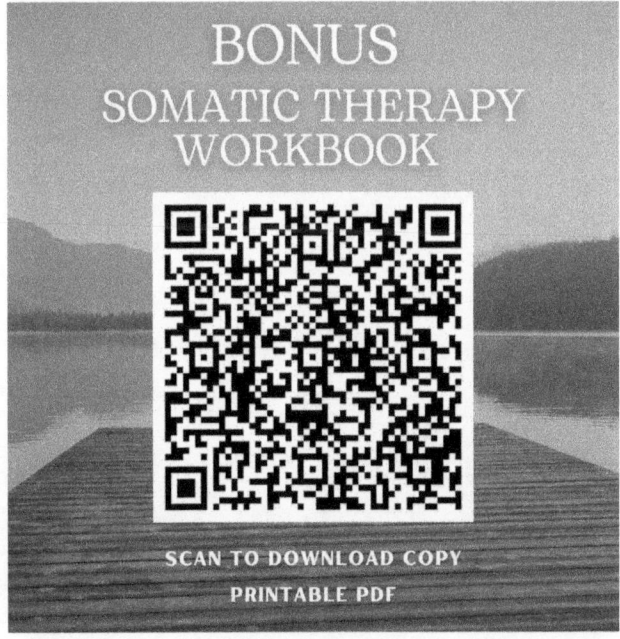

REFERENCES

1 National Center for Biotechnology Information. (n.d.). Somatic experiencing – effectiveness and key factors of a .... Retrieved from https://www.ncbi.nlm.nih.gov/pmc/articles/PMC8276649/

2 Somatic Experiencing International. (n.d.). Somatic experiencing: Supporting trauma resolution and .... Retrieved from https://traumahealing.org/

3 van der Kolk, B. (n.d.). Bessel van der Kolk, MD.: Best-selling trauma research author. Retrieved from https://www.besselvanderkolk.com/

4 Lyon, I. (2016, April 6). 10 practices for creating a safe space in your mind-body .... Retrieved from https://irenelyon.com/2016/04/06/10-practices-creating-safe-space-mind-body-classes/

5 Psych Central. (n.d.). 4 somatic therapy exercises for healing from trauma. Retrieved from https://psychcentral.com/lib/somatic-therapy-exercises-for-trauma

6 Planet Fitness. (n.d.). The ultimate guide to somatic exercises.

REFERENCES

Retrieved from https://www.planetfitness.com/community/articles/somatic-exercise-guide

7 Greatist. (n.d.). What it actually means to "listen to your body". Retrieved from https://greatist.com/move/listen-to-your-body-fitness

8 Somatic Movement Center. (n.d.). How to get rid of your chronic neck pain: Pandiculate!. Retrieved from https://somaticmovementcenter.com/neck-pain/

9 Somatic Movement Center. (n.d.). Somatics exercise for back pain - Learn at home. Retrieved from https://somaticmovementcenter.com/somatics-exercise-for-back-pain/

10 Somatic Movement Center. (n.d.). Relieve neck & shoulder tension with pandiculation. Retrieved from https://somaticmovementcenter.com/neck-and-shoulder-tension/

11 Yoga with Rachel. (n.d.). Somatic exercises for the hips. Retrieved from https://www.yogawithrachelmarie.com/post/somatic-exercises-for-the-hips

12 Verywell Mind. (n.d.). Grounding techniques for coping with PTSD and anxiety. Retrieved from https://www.verywellmind.com/grounding-techniques-for-ptsd-2797300

13 Othership. (n.d.). Breathwork for healing trauma: 3 popular techniques. Retrieved from https://www.othership.us/resources/breathwork-for-healing-trauma

14 The Nalaverse. (n.d.). How breathwork for trauma recovery can facilitate healing. Retrieved from https://thenalaverse.com/blog/how-breathwork-for-trauma-recovery-can-facilitate-healing

15 Healthline. (n.d.). Body scan meditation: Benefits and how to do it. Retrieved from https://www.healthline.com/health/body-scan-meditation

REFERENCES

16 WebMD. (n.d.). Breathing techniques for stress relief. Retrieved from https://www.webmd.com/balance/stress-management/stress-relief-breathing-techniques

17 Brooklyn Somatic Therapy. (n.d.). Somatic techniques for stress and anxiety. Retrieved from https://www.brooklynsomatictherapy.com/blog/somatic-techniques-for-stress-and-anxiety

18 Life Counseling Institute. (n.d.). 10 daily habits that can reduce your anxiety - Willowbrook. Retrieved from https://lifecounselinginstitute.com/10-daily-habits-that-can-reduce-your-anxiety/

19 Mindful Minutes. (n.d.). Ease anxiety with these 5 visualization techniques. Retrieved from https://mindfulminutes.com/ease-anxiety-with-visualization-techniques

20 National Alliance on Mental Illness. (2017, August). The power of a morning routine. Retrieved from https://www.nami.org/Blogs/NAMI-Blog/August-2017/The-Power-of-a-Morning-Routine

21 National Center for Biotechnology Information. (n.d.). Tai chi exercise for mental and physical well-being in .... Retrieved from https://www.ncbi.nlm.nih.gov/pmc/articles/PMC9957102/

22 National Center for Biotechnology Information. (n.d.). Diaphragmatic breathing exercises in recovery from fatigue .... Retrieved from https://www.ncbi.nlm.nih.gov/pmc/articles/PMC10340528/

23 Healthline. (n.d.). 7 science-based health benefits of drinking enough water. Retrieved from https://www.healthline.com/nutrition/7-health-benefits-of-water

24 Well+Good. (n.d.). 60-second somatic release exercise for stress. Retrieved from https://www.wellandgood.com/somatic-release-exercise/

REFERENCES

25 Johns Hopkins Medicine. (n.d.). Somatic self-care | Office of Well-Being. Retrieved from https://www.hopkinsmedicine.org/office-of-well-being/connection-support/somatic-self-care

26 Compassionify. (n.d.). Somatic exercises for anxiety: Relieve stress and tension .... Retrieved from https://compassionify.com/somatic-exercises-for-anxiety/

27 Neff, K. (n.d.). Self-compassion and burnout. Retrieved from https://self-compassion.org/blog/self-compassion-and-burnout/

28 Verywell Health. (n.d.). How does deep breathing improve your digestion?. Retrieved from https://www.verywellhealth.com/diaphragmatic-breathing-stress-digestion-5209648

29 Healthline. (n.d.). Can yoga help aid digestion? 9 poses to try. Retrieved from https://www.healthline.com/nutrition/yoga-posture-for-digestion

30 National Center for Biotechnology Information. (n.d.). Exercise influence on the microbiome–gut–brain axis. Retrieved from https://www.ncbi.nlm.nih.gov/pmc/articles/PMC6748614/

31 Somatopia. (n.d.). The mind-gut connection: How your stomach holds .... Retrieved from https://www.somatopia.com/blog/the-mind-gut-connection-how-your-stomach-holds-emotional-keys

32 Calm. (n.d.). Wind-down time: How and why to add it to your daily routine. Retrieved from https://www.calm.com/blog/wind-down-time

33 Hospital for Special Surgery. (n.d.). 10 stretches to do before bed to improve your sleep. Retrieved from https://www.hss.edu/article_stretches-before-bed.asp

34 Healthline. (n.d.). 8 breathing exercises for sleep: Techniques that work. Retrieved from https://www.healthline.com/health/breathing-exercises-for-sleep

REFERENCES

35 Centers for Disease Control and Prevention. (n.d.). Create a good sleep environment. Retrieved from https://www.cdc.gov/niosh/work-hour-training-for-nurses/longhours/mod6/02.html

36 National Center for Biotechnology Information. (n.d.). Breathe—Your immune system is counting on it. Retrieved from https://www.ncbi.nlm.nih.gov/pmc/articles/PMC7970320/

37 EatingWell. (n.d.). 5 exercises you can do at home to reduce inflammation. Retrieved from https://www.eatingwell.com/article/7677835/5-exercises-you-can-do-at-home-to-reduce-inflammation/

38 National Center for Biotechnology Information. (n.d.). Impact of yoga on inflammatory biomarkers: A systematic .... Retrieved from https://www.ncbi.nlm.nih.gov/pmc/articles/PMC6700894/

39 Harvard Health Publishing. (n.d.). How to boost your immune system. Retrieved from https://www.health.harvard.edu/staying-healthy/how-to-boost-your-immune-system

40 StatPearls. (n.d.). Neuroanatomy, cranial nerve 10 (vagus nerve). Retrieved from https://www.ncbi.nlm.nih.gov/books/NBK537171/

41 Counselling Directory. (n.d.). Polyvagal exercises: A path to reducing stress and chronic .... Retrieved from https://www.counselling-directory.org.uk/memberarticles/polyvagal-exercises-a-path-to-reducing-stress-and-chronic-pain

42 Parsley Health. (n.d.). 8 vagus nerve stimulation exercises that help you relax. Retrieved from https://www.parsleyhealth.com/blog/how-to-stimulate-vagus-nerve-exercises

43 Mayo Clinic. (n.d.). Vagus nerve stimulation. Retrieved from https://www.mayoclinic.org/tests-procedures/vagus-nerve-stimulation/about/pac-20384565

REFERENCES

44 PositivePsychology.com. (n.d.). What is nervous system regulation & why is it important?. Retrieved from https://positivepsychology.com/nervous-system-regulation/

45 Cleveland Clinic. (n.d.). Diaphragmatic breathing exercises & benefits. Retrieved from https://my.clevelandclinic.org/health/articles/9445-diaphragmatic-breathing

46 Cleveland Clinic. (n.d.). 5 ways to stimulate your vagus nerve. Retrieved from https://health.clevelandclinic.org/vagus-nerve-stimulation

47 Canyon Vista Recovery Center. (n.d.). Activating the parasympathetic nervous system. Retrieved from https://canyonvista.com/blog/activating-parasympathetic-nervous-system/

48 Yoga with Rachel. (n.d.). Explore internal sensations with somatic yoga. Retrieved from https://www.yogawithrachelmarie.com/post/somatic-yoga

49 Total Somatics. (n.d.). How to increase productivity with the total somatics approach to health and well-being. Retrieved from https://totalsomatics.com/how-to-increase-productivity-with-the-total-somatics-approach-to-health-and-well-being/

50 Integrative Psychology. (n.d.). 10 somatic interventions explained. Retrieved from https://integrativepsych.co/new-blog/somatic-therapy-explained-methods

51 Psychotherapy.net. (n.d.). Peter Levine on trauma healing: A somatic approach. Retrieved from https://www.psychotherapy.net/interview/interview-peter-levine

52 PositivePsychology.com. (n.d.). Somatic experiencing therapy: 10 best exercises & .... Retrieved from https://positivepsychology.com/somatic-experiencing/

www.ingramcontent.com/pod-product-compliance
Lightning Source LLC
Chambersburg PA
CBHW031156020426
42333CB00013B/694